AF675658

ScyMed™

MediCalc.com™

ScyMed

MediCalc.com™

Medical Calculator System™

MediCalc.com™ *Companion Manual* (1st edition)

MediCalc™ *on line edition* (beta version)

1999

A. Arturo Rodriguez, MD

SCYMED, SA de CV

Mexico City 14000

ScyMed™

MediCalc.com™

MediCalc.com™ *Companion Manual* (1st edition)

MediCalc™ *on-Line edition* (beta version)

A. ARTURO RODRIGUEZ, MD, MBA
The University of Chicago, GSB; Chicago, IL
Internal Medicine, University of Connecticut Health Science Center; Farmington, CT

SCYMED, SA de CV
Apdo Postal (PO Box): 22-922
Mexico City 14000

http://scymed.com

ISBN 968-6277-51-X

 PADLCH 0 1 1 2 3 5 8 13

PRINTED IN USA

This book is dedicated to

Paola

my companion in life
(and wife)

San Diego, Ca. Summer 1998

PREFACE

<< Science is measurement >>................. **HELMHOLTZ**

The application of information technology to medicine is as complex as exciting. The MediCalc™ System is the product of a fine harmonization, integration and synthesis of many different disciplines. From medicine itself, to software, the internet, java and html, www, computing, info tech, etc. The system 'pairs' this *companion manual* and the *MediCalc™ on-line edition*. It features a unique "on-Line, interactive, real time Medical Calculator System™", without a doubt, one of the most innovative clinical tools in medicine.

This manual is the most complete and up-to-date compendium of medical formulas and equations commonly used in clinical practice. Formulas in the manual have their own *formula page™* counterparts on the on-line version (website) and the Medical Calculator System™ performs the computations automatically, reliably and accurately.

My team has made a tremendous effort to assure that notation (medical & arithmetical) as well as information are current and accurate. The on-Line Medical Calculator System™ has been extensively tested and will continue beta-testing, so that potential errors and bugs can be corrected. Users are encouraged to be very careful in selecting and interpreting clinical data, inputs and output results. Furthermore, they are warned to always check computations manually.

I am sure that MediCalc™ will facilitate -and standardize- clinical quantitative data analysis and the learning and reasoning processes involved. My main objective, in one sentence, is to help physicians manage and process clinical information more efficiently and consequently, improve the quality of care.

I am grateful to the many Colleagues, Programmers, tech personnel and friends who collaborated (and continue to do so) in the exciting development of the MediCalc™ project.

Comments and suggestions are welcome, email to:
arturo.rodriguez@gsbalum.uchicago.edu or
feedback@medicalc.com

AAR

REGISTRATION

- Purchase of this manual includes a **2-week FREE TRIAL** of the on-line edition (unlimited access), also, you get a credit for **$20 dollars** towards the annual subscription.

- *THIS OFFER IS FOR INDIVIDUALS ONLY.*

Check our website for exact dates and promotions.
*certain restrictions apply, offer subject to change without notice.

- **To activate access (Free trial) you need:**

1.- The password (follow instructions at the website).

2.- Agree with the terms of Use and email us the short application form (www.medicalc.com/registry/form.htm)

3.- Keep your sales receipt (proof of purchase).

Visit our website at: **http://www.MediCalc.com**

SYSTEM REQUIREMENTS for on-line use

- **1.-** IBM compatible PC (mouse and keyboard). (200MHz processor or higher, 32MB of RAM/higher).

2.- 28.8K Modem (or faster).

3.- WWW browser (microsoft Internet explorer 4.0/higher).

4.- Internet access.

- **NOTICE:**

The MediCalc™ on-line edition and the on-Line Medical Calculator System™ have only been tested on IBM compatible PCs running Microsoft Internet Explorer 4.0 & windows95.

Apdo Postal (P.O. Box): 22-922
Mexico City 14000

NOTICE

IMPORTANT (read carefully): Most of the clinical formulas were devised under strict conditions, they have to be taken "**only**" as guidelines, not the "last word", assumptions must be carefully considered and the original sources must be consulted routinely. Normal Values vary between Laboratories, it is essential to check the normal values of the Laboratory performing the test.

The package insert for each drug should be consulted routinely for use and dosage prior to prescription and/or administration.

DISCLAIMER

IMPORTANT (read carefully): In using MediCalc™, Physicians and other healthcare professionals, have the sole responsibility to be fully aware of current medical and clinical practices and standards, to employ good clinical judgement in selecting and interpreting clinical data (input and output results), **and to verify all calculations obtained through the use of the MediCalc™ on-line edition manually**. The beta version of the on-line edition software IS NOT INTENDED FOR DIRECT PATIENT CARE but rather for teaching and research activities. The system is being tested (beta version) and errors and bugs are possible. Users are also encouraged to confirm the information contained herein and/or the on-line edition with other sources. This recommendation is of particular importance in connection with infrequently used medical information.

ScyMed, SA de CV ("ScyMed") makes no warranty whatsoever, expressed or implied, including any warranty as to accuracy, completeness or timeliness, concerning the information, views and/or functionality available or obtained at or through the use of the MediCalc™ manual and/or the on-line edition.

ScyMed shall not be liable to you or anyone else in any way for any loss, claim or damages.

Physicians and Healthcare professionals with comments or questions about MediCalc™ should e-mail us at:
info@MediCalc.com

Thank You!

ScyMed, SA de CV, Mexico City 14000

CONTENTS

Contents (cont)

on-Line CONTENTS

MediCalc™ on-line **Contents**

on-Line Medical Calculator System™

Formula-pages™ (Formulas & Equations):

Formula-page™ complete internet (website) address:

e.g. http://www.medicalc.com/frmls/directory/document.htm

(e.g for HR = http://www.medicalc.com/frmls/hemodyn/HR.htm)

MediCalc™ on-line

Formula-page™ complete internet (website) address:

e.g. http://www.medicalc.com/frmls/directory/document.htm

(e.g. for VD = http://www.medicalc.com/frmls/pulmo/VD.htm)

/frmls **/directory** **/document.htm**

/pulmo

on-Line Contents

	/frmls	/directory			/document.htm
		/renal			

MediCalc™ on-line

Formula-page™ complete internet (website) address:

		/frmls	/directory	/document.htm
			/renal	

RENAL (cont)

NUTRITION

		/frmls	/directory	/document.htm
			/nutrition	

on-Line Contents

MediCalc™ on-line edition Contents

Formula-page™ complete internet (website) address:

	/frmls	/directory	/document.htm
		/conversion	

CONVERSION

* The internet address of the Formulas is also included in this manual (e.g for HR, see page 7 and follow the icon).

NOTICE: The arrow ▸ indicates that the formula-page™ will be accessible on-Line by september 24, 1998. The rest will be implemented at the discretion of ScyMed, SA de CV. in the following weeks.

Website contents and function subject to change without notice.

Login Instructions

To login to the MediCalc™ on-line edition you need:

1.- Your user name and password.

2.- The complete internet address of the formula-page™ *.

3.- A Computer with keyboard and mouse, internet access and a WWW browser (MS internet explorer 4.0/higher).

IMPORTANT (read carefully):

MediCalc™ on-line edition is in a Beta testing period, some Formula-pages™ won't be hyperlinked in this version. This means that Users can only access the pages by typing in the complete internet address on the web browser *address field.* Hyperlinks will be implemmented in the following versions depending on Users' practices, demand and availability.

... find more about this at http://www.medicalc.com

▸ *never give your user name or password to anybody.*

CARDIAC FUNCTION

Hemodynamics

HR Heart Rate — 60 - 80 bpm

HR = C.O. (1000mL) / SV

http://www.medicalc.com/frmls/hemodyn/**HR.htm**

SV Stroke Volume — 78 ± 9 mL/beat [*a]

SV = C.O. (1000mL) / HR

http://www.medicalc.com/frmls/hemodyn/**SV.htm**

SVI Stroke Volume Index — 46 ± 5 mL/beat/m2

SVI = C.I. (1000mL) / HR

http://www.medicalc.com/frmls/hemodyn/**SVI.htm**

CO Cardiac Output — 5.4 L/min

Fick Equation:

$$C.O. = \frac{VO_2}{C(a\text{-}v)O_2}$$

http://www.medicalc.com/frmls/hemodyn/**CO_fick.htm**

Physiologic:

C.O. = HR * SV

http://www.medicalc.com/frmls/hemodyn/**CO_phys.htm**

CI Cardiac Index — 2.5 - 4.0 L/min/m2

CI = C.O. / BSA

http://www.medicalc.com/frmls/hemodyn/**CI.htm**

MTT	Mean Transit Time	15 ± 1.4 s
EDV	End-Diastolic Volume	75 ± 15 mL/m2
ESV	End-Systolic Volume	25 ± 8 mL/m2
EF	Ejection Fraction	0.67 (0.55 - 0.78)

EF = SV / EDV

http://www.medicalc.com/frmls/hemodyn/**EF.htm**

*a : value for 1.7m2 of BSA. *b : PV= plasma volume.

Hemodynamics

BV	Blood Volume BV = PV / (1 – Hct) * BSA	2.37 L/m2 (F) [*b] 2.74 L/m2 (M)
	http://www.medicalc.com/frmls/hemodyn/**BV.htm**	
CBVI	Central Blood Volume Index CBVI = MTT * CI * 16.7	830 ± 86 mL/m2
	http://www.medicalc.com/frmls/hemodyn/**CBVI.htm**	
BFVR	Blood Flow Volume Ratio BFVR = CI / BVI	1.2 (F) 1.1 (M)
	http://www.medicalc.com/frmls/hemodyn/**BFVR.htm**	
CBF	Cerebral Blood Flow CBF = (MAP – ICP) / CVR	50-60mL/min/100g tissue [*c]
MBF	Myocardial Blood Flow MBF = (MAP – PRA) / CVR	60mL/min/100g tissue [*d]
RBF	Renal Blood Flow, basal	25% of C.O.

Circulation Times

Arm to Lung (ether)	2 - 12 s
Arm to Tongue (Ca gluconate)	12 - 18 s
Arm to Tongue (Decholin)	10 - 16 s

CONTRACTILITY

Maximum Left Ventricular dp/dt	1650±300 mmHg/s
Maximum (dp/dt)/p	44 ± 8.4 s^{-1}
(dp/dt)/DP (at DP= 40mmHg)	37.6 ± 12.2 s^{-1}
Systolic Ejection rate (mean, norm)	3.32 ± 0.84EDV/s
Circumferential Fiber Shortening Mean Velocity of (angiography)	1.66±0.42circumf/s

* b : PV = plasma volume. * c : CVR = cerebro-vascular resistance.
* d : CVR = coronary vascular resistance.

Hemodynamics

CARDIAC WORK

LCWI Left Cardiac Work Index 3.8 ± 0.4 kg*m/m2
LCWI = CI * MAP * 0.0144
http://www.medicalc.com/frmls/hemodyn/**LCWI.htm**

RCWI Right Cardiac Work Index 0.6 ± 0.06 kg*m/m2
RCWI = CI * MPAP * 0.0144
http://www.medicalc.com/frmls/hemodyn/**RCWI.htm**

LVSWI Left Vent Stroke Work Index 56 ± 6 g*m/m2
LVSWI= SI * MAP * 0.0144
http://www.medicalc.com/frmls/hemodyn/**LVSWI.htm**

RVSWI Right vent stroke work index 8.8 ± 0.9 g*m/m2
RVSWI SI * MPAP * 0.0144
http://www.medicalc.com/frmls/hemodyn/**RVSWI.htm**

*0.0144 is a conversion term to equalize units

RESISTANCES

SVR Systemic Vascular Resistance 770-1500dyn*s/cm5
SVR = ((MAP – CVP) * 79.92) / C.O.
http://www.medicalc.com/frmls/hemodyn/**SVR.htm**

SVRI Systemic Vasc Resist Index 2180±210dyn*s/cm5/m2
SVRI = ((MAP – CVP) * 79.92) / C.I.
http://www.medicalc.com/frmls/hemodyn/**SVRI.htm**

PVR Pulmonary Vascular Resistance 20-120dyn*s/cm5
PVR = ((MPAP – WP) * 79.92) / C.O.
http://www.medicalc.com/frmls/hemodyn/**PVR.htm**

PVRI Pulmonary Vasc Resist Index 270±15dyn*s/cm5/m2
PVRI = ((MPAP – WP) * 79.92) / C.I.
http://www.medicalc.com/frmls/hemodyn/**PVRI.htm**

*79.92 is a conversion term to equalize units

* Cardiac work formulas can be unindexed multiplying indexed parameters by BSA (e.g. LCW= LCWI * BSA), alternatively, CI or SI may be used instead of C.O. or SV.

Pressures

MAP Mean Arterial Pressure — 93 (70-105) mmHg

$$MAP = \frac{(SP + 2DP)}{3}$$

http://www.medicalc.com/frmls/hemodyn/**MAP.htm**

MPAP Mean Pulmonary Arterial Press. — 5 – 10 mmHg

$$MPAP = \frac{(PAS + 2PAD)}{3}$$

http://www.medicalc.com/frmls/hemodyn/**MPAP.htm**

RPP Rate Pressure Product — < 12,000

RPP = HR * SAP

http://www.medicalc.com/frmls/hemodyn/**RPP.htm**

PP Pulse Pressure — ~ 40 mmHg

PP = SP – DP

http://www.medicalc.com/frmls/hemodyn/**PP.htm**

COP Colloid-Oncotic Pressure — 25 mmHg

COP = (1.4 * globulin) + (5.5 * albumin)

albumin and globulin in g/dL in serum.

http://www.medicalc.com/frmls/hemodyn/**COP.htm**

Goldman equation (myocardial irritability)

$$GE = \frac{(K+)(Mg+)(H+)}{(Na+)(Ca++)}$$

* MAP and MPAP can also be computed as: MAP= SP + 0.33(SP – DP). and MPAP= PAS + 0.33(PAS – PAD). (use 0.33 or 1/3).

Pressures

Pressure	systolic	diastolic	mean
BP, SAP	120	80	93
Left Ventricle	120	0 – 12	
Left Atria	10	12	10
WP	10	12	10
PAP	25	12	16
Right Ventricle	25	0 – 6	
Right Atria	6	6	4
CVP	-2 insp	+4 exp (cmH2O)	

*all pressures in mmHg, unless otherwise stated.
BP= blood pressure. SAP= systemic arterial pressure.
WP= wedge pressure (also called PAOP= pulm artery oclussion pressure).
PAP= pulmonary arterial pressure. CVP= central venous pressure.

Portal Vein Pressure

nl= 10 – 15 cmH2O (7-10mmHg)
portal htn= > 30 cmH2O (saline)

	plasma	venous	interstitial
Oncotic	25 ± 2	26 ± 2	15 - 20

capillary	arterial	venous	tissue
Hydrostatic	30 ± 5	10 – 15	0 – 2

*all pressures in mmHg.

Hemodynamic Patterns

Condition	SAP	CVP	PAP	PCWP	C.O.	C(a–v)O_2	PVR	SVR
Hypovolemic shock	↓	↓	↓	↓	↓	↑	→↑	↑
Cardiogenic shock	↓	↑	↑	↑	↓	↑	→↑	↑
Septic shock (distributive)	↓	↓	↓	↓	↑	↓	→↓	↓
Cardiac tamponade	↓	↑	↑	↑	↓	↑	→	↑
Right Ventricle Infarction	↓	↑	→	→	↓	↑	→	→↑
Pulmonary embolism (obstructive)	↓	↑	↑	→↓	↓	↑	↑	↑
Airways obstruction	→↓	→↑	↑	→	→↓	→	↑	→

↓= decrease. ↑= increase. →= normal. SAP= systolic arterial pressure. CVP= central venous pressure. PAP= pulmonary arterial pressure. PCWP= pulmonary capillary wedge pressure. C.O.= cardiac output. C(a-v)O2 = arterial-venous O2 content difference. PVR= pulmonary vascular resistance. SVR= systemic vascular resistance. SOURCE: Modified from references in CardioPulmonary/Hemodynamics.

ElectroCardioGraphy

Axis

QRS: nl = –30° → +100°

Left Axis Deviation= –30° → –90°

(normal variation, emphysema, RVH, RBBB, WPW)

Right Axis Deviation= +100° → +180°

–90° → –180°

(normal variation, mechanical shifts, LAH, LBBB, WPW, emphysema)

P Wave = +30° → +60°

Assess: I and AVF, then find isoelectric lead and QRS axis is at 90°.

QRS:	**Lead I**	**Lead AVF**
extreme RAD	–	–
Right Axis deviation	–	+
normal range	+	+
Left Axis deviation	+	–

HEXAXIAL SYSTEM

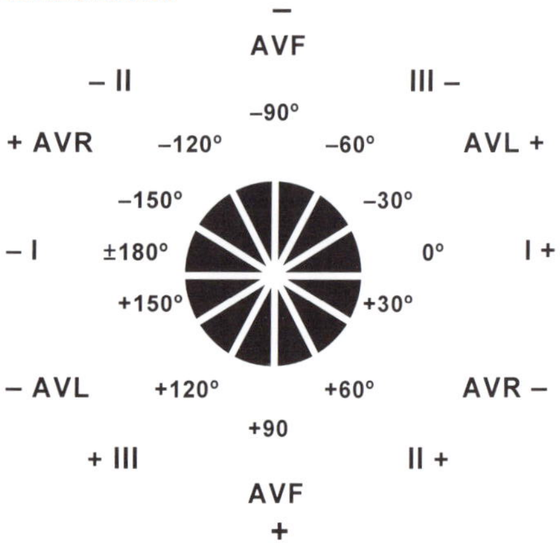

Rate ECG

HR by small box	mm
300	**5**
250	6
214	7
187	8
167	9
150	**10**
136	11
125	12
115	13
107	14
100	**15**
94	16
88	17
83	18
79	19
75	**20**
71	21
68	22
65	23
63	24
60	**25**
58	26
56	27
54	28
52	29
50	**30**
43	**35**
38	**40**
33	**45**
30	**50**
27	**55**
25	**60**
23	**65**
20	**75**
15	**100**

Normal HR = 80 ± 20 bpm
EKG Paper speed = 25mm/sec
small box = 0.04 sec = 1mm
large box = 0.20 sec = 5mm

estimate HR
correlate number of boxes with fig on the left
Heart Rate = (1500 / # of small boxes)

Pacemakers:
SA Node = 60 -100/min
Atrium = 75/min
AV Node = 40 - 60/min
Ventricular = 30 - 40/min

Waveforms & Intervals

P= < 0.10s, ↑ I, II; ↓ AVR
PR= 0.12 - 0.20s
QRS= 0.05 - 0.10s
anterior leads height: <27mm
↑ I, II, V5, V6
↓ AVR, V1
↑↓ V3, AVL, AVF, III
T= ↑ I, V6; ↓ AVR;
may invert: III, AVF, AVL, V1
Q Wave (abnormal)=
> 0.04s, > 25% of height of following R
QT= 0.34s - 0.42s (40% of R-R)
(↑ HR → ↓ QT)
60 bpm = 0.33 - 0.43 s
70 bpm = 0.31 - 0.41 s
80 bpm = 0.29 - 0.38 s
90 bpm = 0.28 - 0.36 s
100 bpm = 0.27 - 0.35 s

http://www.medicalc.com/frmls/ekg/QT_c.htm

QT (corrected) = $\frac{QT}{\sqrt{R\text{-}R\ (s)}}$

Rhythms

NSR= Normal Sinus Rhytm
(60 – 100 beats/min), stable P-P, R-R intervals.
Sinus Tach = > 100/min.
Sinus Brad = < 60/min.

APD= (atrial premature depolarization).
preceded by P wave, followed by nl QRS.

VPD= (vent premature depolarization).
premature QRS >0.12s.
no P wave, T wave is large, opposite to QRS.
(in nl subjects and Heart Dz).
Multifocal PVC's= diff PVC's in same strip.

PAT= (paroxysmal atrial tachycardia).
Identifiable P, narrow QRS, 150-250/min.

MAT= (multifocal atrial tachycardia).
≥ 3 diff ectopic P waves, varying
PR, nl QRS, 100-200/min.
in COPD, hypoxia, digitalis, ASHD,
aminophyline intox.

SVT= (supraventricular tachycardia).
150-250/min. QRS usually normal.
wide QRS with BBB or WPW.

a) AV Node Reentry:
retrograde P buried in QRS.
RP <50% RR interval.

b) Orthodromic SVT with acc path:
eccentric, retrograde P wave
RP <50%RR interval.
Negative P wave in I.

c) Intra-atrial reentry:
+ P wave in leads II, III, AVF.
RP >50% RR interval.

d) Sinus Node reentry:
P wave same as sinus rhythm.
RP >50% RR interval.

e) Automatic Atrial Tach:
↑ or ↓ P wave in II,III, AVF.
RP >50% RR interval.

Atrial Flutter=
atrial rate 240-350/min.
Ventricular rate varies with AV block 2:1
Saw tooth pattern (II, III, AVF, V1).

Atrial Fib= Highly irregular, irregular.
No P waves.
Ventricular response: 160-200/min.

Bigeminy= coupled beat.
sinus beat→PVC→sinus beat→ PVC

Trigeminy=
sinus→sinus→PVC →sinus→sinus→PVC
Ectopic Escapes= follow sinus pause.

V Tach= (ventricular tachycardia).
≥ 3 wide QRS (≥0.12s) rate: 100-250/min.
ST and T wave change direction.
AV dissociation, LAD, RBBB.
Sustained (>30s), or non-sustained.

Torsades de Pointes=
is a kind of V tach. 160-280/min.
twisting of QRS, prolonged QT.

V Fib= (ventricular fibrillation).
very irregular baseline
with cardiac arrest and Blood Pressure = 0

AIVR= (accelerated idioventricular rhythm).
Rate: 50-100/min
wide QRS (in inferior wall MI).

Hypertrophy

RAH= (Right Atrial Hypertrophy)
Diphasic tall initial component of P wave > 2.5mm in II
(P pulmonale, also in III, AVF)

LAH= (Left Atrial Hypertrophy)
Diphasic P wave with wide terminal
component in V1. P ≥ 0.12s.
P mitrale- wide
M-shaped P in I, II, AVF.

RVH= (Right Ventricular Hypertrophy)
RAD >+100°, incomplete RBBB V1
R ≥ S in V1. R > 5mm in V1
Decreasing R wave V1→ V4
RV strain pattern = ST depression and ↓ T's V1→V3

LVH= (Left Ventricular Hypertrophy)
LAH. LAD without LBBB or LAHB
S (V1 or V2) **+ R** (V5 or V6) = ≥ 35 mm
R in V5 or V6 > 25mm
LV strain pattern = ± ST depression + ↓T's
(I II, III, AVL or AVF, V5, V6)
R AVL ≥ 12mm. R AVF ≥ 20mm

Ischemia

Ischemia = flat or inverted T waves
Injury & Infarct = ST seg. ↑ or ↓
Infarction= q wave > 0.04s (acute/old)
(tiny Q waves in I, II, AVL, V5, V6)
LBBB complicates diagnosis of MI

Location	Leads	Vessels
Anterior	V2-V4	LAD
Anteroseptal	V1-V4	LAD
Anterolateral	V1,V6,I,AVL	LAD, Diagonal
Inferior	II, III, AVF	RCA, Circumflex
Lateral	I,AVL,V5-V6	Circumflex, Diagonal
Posterior	tall R= V1-V3	RCA
Right Ventricle	right V4	RCA

Heart Blocks ECG

1° AV Block=

PR interval > 0.20s
All P's associated with QRS

2° AV Block=

Type I = Mobitz I, Wenckebach (AV Node Dysfunction)
PR interval ↑ until QRS is dropped.
usually 3:2, 4:3, 5:4.

Type II = Mobitz II (Infra His Dysfunction)
PR interval constant until QRS is dropped.

3° AV Block=

Complete AV Block=
No AV conduction.
P has no relation to QRS.
Slow ventricular escape rhythm
stable P-P intervals

RBBB = Right Bundle Branch Block
QRS > 0.12s
Deep and round S waves in leads I, AVL, V4 - V6
RR' or M pattern of QRS in leads V1 - V3
S-T, T wave changes in V1-V3

LBBB = Left Bundle Branch Block
QRS > 0.12s
No septal Q in V4-V6, I, AVL
RR' or M pattern of QRS and S-T,
T wave Changes in leads I, AVL, V4 - V6

Anterior Hemiblock=
LAD (– 60°)
QRS 0.10 - 0.12s
small Q in I, AVL
R in II, III and AVF
terminal R in AVR

Posterior Hemiblock=
RAD (+ 120°)
QRS 0.10 - 0.12s
S in I
Q in II, III and AVF

specific EKG changes

Pericarditis =
ST ↑ (precordial leads)
± ↓ voltage, ± ↓ T waves

COPD =
RAD (– lead I) ↓ voltage
P pulmonale (RAH)
± RBBB

Pulmonary Embolism, Infarct =
S in I, Q in III ; S1 Q3 T3
Sinus Tachycardia
RAD, ± RBBB
variable ST and T changes

Hyperthyroidism =
Sinus Tachycardia

Hypothyroidism =
Sinus Bradycardia, ↓ voltage
ST depression
flat or ↓ T waves

Hypothermia (systemic) **=**
Prolongs repolarization
Osborn wave:
convex ↑ of J point

Intracraneal Bleed
(severe) =
QT prolongation
T wave ↓
(Subarachnoid Hemorrhage).

↑ K^+ (hyperkalemia) =
T waves: peaked, tenting
P wave: wide → flat
QRS: wide
QT interval widening
Sine Waves → Asystole

↓ K^+ (hypokalemia) =
flat T waves, U wave (U > T)
ST depression

↑ Ca^{++} (hypercalcemia) =
Short QT.

↓ Ca^{++} (hypocalcemia) =
Prolonged QT (ST portion).

Digoxin =
nl: shorter QT + downward curve of ST segment and flat or ↓ T waves.
Toxicity: SA block, AV Block, junctional TC, PVC's, Bi- & Trigeminy, V Tach, V Fib.

Quinidine =
P: wide, notched.
QRS: wide.
ST segment ↓.
QT: prolonged.
U wave.

Tricyclics OD =
QRS and QT prolongation
Sinus Tachycardia

* ↑ = increased or elevated. ↓ = decreased, depressed or inverted.

PULMONARY

Lung Volumes

RR	Respiratory rate	**12 – 16 /min**
TV **VT**	Tidal Volume TV = IC – IRV (volume inspired/expired with each breath)	**0.5 L** (7–15 ml/Kg)
TLC	Total Lung Capacity TLC = VC + RV (volume in the lungs at maximal inspiration)	**6.0 L (± 1.0)**
VC	Vital Capacity VC = IRV + TV + ERV (max volume expelled by forceful effort after max inspiration) Sex: F = 50-60mL/Kg. M = 70mL/Kg.	**4.5 L (± 0.5)**
IC	Inspiratory Capacity IC = IRV + TV (maximum volume inspired from resting expiration)	**3.0 L (± 1.0)**
IRV	Inspiratory Reserve Volume IRV = IC – TV (maximal inspired volume from end-tidal inspiration)	**2.5 L**
ERV	Expiratory Reserve Volume ERV = FRC – RV (maximal expired volume form end-tidal inspiration)	**1.5 L (± 0.5)** 25% of VC
FRC	Functional Residual Capacity FRC = ERV + RV (volume in lungs after tidal volume is expired)	**3.0 L (± 1.0)**
RV	Residual Volume RV = FRC – ERV (volume in lungs after maximal expiration)	**1.5 L (± 0.5)**

http://www.medicalc.com/frmls/pulmo/LungVols.htm

Lung Volumes

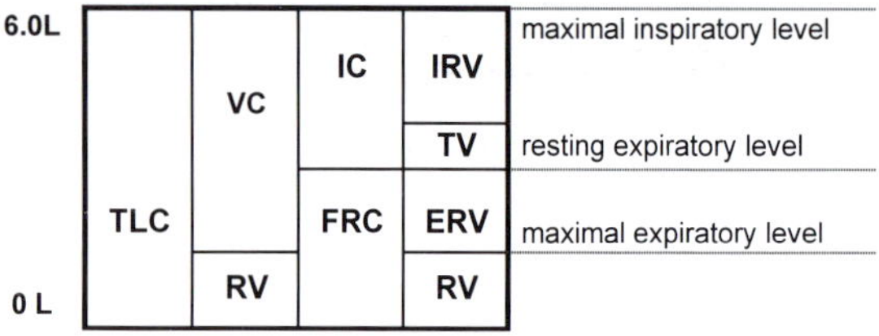

RV/TLC	ratio (> 30% means overdistension)	**25% (<30%)**
CV	Closing Volume	**400 mL**
CV/VC	ratio	**9%**
CC	Closing Capacity CC = CV + RV Increased: age, uremia, cirrhosis, smoking, MI. Decreased: supine, obesity, post-Op, anesthesia, pregnancy.	**1.9 L**
CC/TLC	ratio	**32%**
$\mathbf{V_A}$	Alveolar Volume	**same as FRC**
$\mathbf{V_D}$	Volume of Dead Space	**150 mL** F<M

$$V_D = \frac{V_T\,(PaCO_2 - P\bar{E}CO_2)}{Pa\,CO_2}$$

http://www.medicalc.com/frmls/pulmo/**VD.htm**

Estimated: 1 mL per Lb of Body weight.
Anatomic: conducting airways.
Physiologic: (alveolar), due to V/Q mismatch.

$\mathbf{V_D/V_T}$	Dead Space/Tidal volume ratio Fraction of each V_T not involved in gas exchange.	**0.25 – 0.35**

$$V_D/V_T = \frac{(PaCO_2 - P\bar{E}CO_2)}{Pa\,CO_2}$$

http://www.medicalc.com/frmls/pulmo/**VDVT.htm**

< 0.30 rest. < 0.20 exercise. COPD = 0.4 – 0.5
If > 0.6 may need ventilatory support.

* VD refers to volume of dead space.

Ventilation — PULMONARY

$\dot{V}_E$ Minute Ventilation **6.0 L/min**

(Total volume exhaled per minute).

$\dot{V}_E = (0.863 * \dot{V}CO_2) / [PaCO_2 (1 - V_D/V_T)]$

http://www.medicalc.com/frmls/pulmo/**VEdot.htm**

$\dot{V}_E = V_T * RR, \ (\dot{V}_A + \dot{V}_D)$

estimated= 90mL/Kg/min (↑ 5% per ↑ 1°F)

$\dot{V}_A$ Alveolar Ventilation **4.0 L/min**

(Total gas reaching gas exchange units per min).

$\dot{V}_A = \dot{V}_T - \dot{V}_D$

http://www.medicalc.com/frmls/pulmo/**VAdot.htm**

$\dot{V}_D$ Dead Space Ventilation **2.0 L/min** (<30% $\dot{V}_E$)

(Total volume ventilating the airways, non-perfused lung units, and the ventilation tubing).

$$\dot{V}_D = \frac{\dot{V}_E (PaCO_2 - P\bar{E}CO_2)}{Pa\ CO_2}$$

http://www.medicalc.com/frmls/pulmo/**VDdot.htm**

$\dot{V}_A/Q$ $\dot{V}_A$/Blood Flow **0.8**

Single Breath N_2 Test:

ΔN_2 from 750 to 1250mL in expired gas	<1.5% N_2
Slope of Phase III	<2% N_2/L
Alveolar N_2 after 7 min of breathing O_2	<2.5% N_2

Control of Ventilation

Ventilatory response to hypercapnia	>0.5L/min/torr
Ventilatory response to hypoxia	>0.2L/min ΔSO_2 (%)

Diffusion

Diffusing Capacity for Carbon Monoxide:

DL_{COsb} **32 mL CO/min/torr**

* V = volume. $\dot{V}$ = ventilation

Hemodynamics

$\dot{Q}S$	Shunted Blood R → L, (V/Q = 0) IntraPulmonary: 150mL/min (2 - 3% of CO) Pulmonary AV fistula: Intrapulmonary / HHT* Intracardiac (congenital): VSD, ASD, PDA	**150 mL**
$\dot{Q}T$	Pulmonary Blood Flow Pulmonary capillary blood flow	**5.4 L/min** (4.0-8.0) **5.4 L/min**
$\dot{Q}S/\dot{Q}T$	Shunt Fraction R → L	**< 5%**

$$\dot{Q}S/\dot{Q}T = \frac{CcO_2 - CaO_2}{CcO_2 - C\bar{v}O_2}$$

* ScO_2 assumed to be 1.0

$$\dot{Q}S/\dot{Q}T = \frac{(0.0031)\,(A\text{–}a\dot{D}O_2)}{(0.0031)\,(A\text{–}a\dot{D}O2) + (CaO_2 - C\bar{v}O_2)}$$

http://www.medicalc.com/frmls/pulmo/**QSQT.htm**

Pulmonary Capillary Blood Volume	100 mL
Pulmonary Artery Pressure	15-30 / 5-13mmHg
Pulmonary Capillary Wedge Pressure	2 – 12 mmHg

Gases

FIO_2	Fraction of Inspired O_2	**0.21** (room air)
$F\bar{E}O_2$	Fraction of Expired O_2	**0.17**
$\dot{V}O_2$	Oxygen Consumption $\dot{V}O_2 = \dot{Q}T * C(a\text{–}\bar{v})O_2$	**240mL/min** (STPD*)

http://www.medicalc.com/frmls/pulmo/**VO2.htm**

$\dot{V}O_2I$	Oxygen Consumption Index $\dot{V}O_2I = \dot{V}O_2 / BSA$	**120-160mL/min/m2**

http://www.medicalc.com/frmls/pulmo/**VO2I.htm**

* STPD: Standard conditions: Temperature 0°C, Pressure 760 torr, and dry (0 torr water vapor).

O_2 ext Oxygen extraction rate **20 – 30%**

$$O_2 \text{ ext} = \frac{C(a-\bar{v})O_2}{CaO_2}$$

http://www.medicalc.com/frmls/pulmo/**O2_ext.htm**

$\dot{D}O_2$ Oxygen Delivery **950-1105mL/min**

$\dot{D}O_2 = CO * CaO_2$

http://www.medicalc.com/frmls/pulmo/**DO2.htm**

$\dot{D}O_2I$ Oxygen Delivery Index **550-650mL/min/m2**

$\dot{D}O_2I = CI * CaO_2$

http://www.medicalc.com/frmls/pulmo/**DO2I.htm**

* O_2 content is multiplied by 10 to equalize units.

$\dot{V}CO_2$ Carbon Dioxide Output **192mL/min** (STPD*)

$\dot{V}CO_2$ = 3.2mL/Kg/min (↑ 7% per ↑ 1°C Temp)

http://www.medicalc.com/frmls/pulmo/**VCO2.htm**

R Respiratory Quotient **0.8**

$$R = \frac{\dot{V}CO_2}{\dot{V}O_2}$$

http://www.medicalc.com/frmls/pulmo/**R.htm**

Carbon Dioxide (CO_2)

$PaCO_2$ arterial CO_2 tension **35-45 mmHg**

$PaO_2 + PaCO2 = \leq$ 150mmHg at sea level on RA.

Hypercapnea (↑ CO2) (hypoventilation):
produces pulmonary vasospasm, respiratory depression, dilation of cerebral vessels, papilledema, acidosis.

Hypocapnea (↓ CO2) (hyperventilation):
causes: anxiety, CNS lesions, fever, ↓BP, gram(–) sepsis, hypoxia, metabolic acidosis, ↑thyroid, pain, PE.

*RA= room air. PE= pulmonary embolism

Gases

P_ACO_2	alveolar CO_2 tension * in general equals $PaCO_2$	**40 mmHg**
$P\bar{v}CO_2$	mixed venous CO_2 tension *draw via Pulmonary artery line.	**40-50 mmHg**
$CaCO_2$	arterial CO_2 content	**23-27 mmol/L**
$P\bar{E}CO_2$	expired CO_2 tension *measure PCO_2 of expired gas in douglas bag	

Oxygen (O_2)

PaO_2 arterial O_2 tension — F_IO_2 0.21 : **95 torr** (80-100); F_IO_2 1.0 : **640 torr**

age correction: 100 – 1/3 age
Posture: sitting = 103.5 – 0.42(age)
supine= 104.2 – 0.35(age)
increased PaO_2 : (?) hyperventilation, ↑FIO_2, artifact.

http://www.medicalc.com/frmls/pulmo/**PaO2.htm**

$P\bar{v}O_2$ mixed venous O_2 tension **35-45 mmHg**

Oxygen/Carbon dioxide	ABGs		$A\text{-}aDO_2$	
	PaO2	PaCO2	0.21	1.0
Alveolar Hypoventilation	↓	↑	N	N
↓ F_IO_2 (high altitude)	↓	↓	N	N
V/Q mismatch (regional)	↓	↑/N/↓	↑	N/↑
Intrapulmonary Shunt (R → L)	↓	N/↓	↑	↑
Impaired Diffusion	↓	N/↓	↑	N
Anatomical Shunt (R → L)	↓	N/↓	↑	↑

* V/Q: ventilation/perfusion.
R = right. L = left.

Oxygen Content

CaO2 arterial O_2 content **17 - 21 mL/dL**

O_2 capacity = (Hb (g) /100mL) * 1.36 mL O_2 per g Hb
O_2 content = O_2 combined (~97%) + O_2 dissolved (~3%)

CaO_2 = (1.36 * Hb * (SaO_2/100)) + 0.0031(PaO2)

http://www.medicalc.com/frmls/pulmo/**CaO2.htm**

C$\bar{v}$O2 mixed venous O_2 content **12 - 15 mL/dL**

$C\bar{v}O_2$ = (1.36 * Hb * ($S\bar{v}O_2$/100)) + 0.0031($P\bar{v}O2$)

http://www.medicalc.com/frmls/pulmo/**CvO2.htm**

C(a-$\bar{v}$)O2 arterial - venous O_2 content difference **4 - 5 mL/dL**

$C(a-\bar{v})O_2 = CaO_2 - C\bar{v}O_2$

http://www.medicalc.com/frmls/pulmo/**CavO2.htm**

CcO2 capillary O_2 content **21 mL/dL**

CcO_2 = (1.36 * Hb * (ScO_2/100)) + 0.0031(PaO2)

http://www.medicalc.com/frmls/pulmo/**CcO2.htm**

Hb = hemoglobin (blood, g/dL).
SaO2 = arterial oxygen saturation (%).
S$\bar{v}$O2 = mixed venous oxygen saturation (%).
ScO2 = capillary oxygen saturation (%).
PaO2 = arterial oxygen tension (mmHg)
P$\bar{v}$O2 = mixed venous oxygen tension (mmHg).

O_2 Therapy	Flow rate L/min	%O_2 delivered*
Nasal Prongs	1	24%
	2	28%
	3	32%
	4	36%
*approximate values	5	40%

*% of O2 delivered increases 3-4% per each 1 liter/min.

A-a Gradient

A a GRADIENT

P_B Barometric pressure (sea level) **760 mmHg**

http://www.medicalc.com/frmls/pulmo/**PB.htm**

PH_2O Water vapor pressure **47 mmHg**

P_IO_2 Inspired O_2 tension **150 mmHg**

$P_IO_2 = F_IO_2 (P_B - PH_2O)$

http://www.medicalc.com/frmls/pulmo/**PIO2.htm**

P_AO_2 alveolar O_2 tension F_IO_2 0.21 : **100 torr**
F_IO_2 1.0 : **673 torr**

$$P_AO_2 = F_IO_2 (P_B - PH_2O) - \frac{PaCO_2}{R}$$

$P_AO_2 = (F_IO_2 * 713) - (PaCO_2 / 0.8)$ at sea level, RA.

http://www.medicalc.com/frmls/pulmo/**PAlvO2.htm**

$A\text{-}a\dot{D}O_2$
$P(A\text{-}a)O_2$ Alveolar-arterial O_2 GRADIENT **5-25mmHg** (FIO_2 0.21)
<150mmHg (FIO_2 1.0)

$$A\text{-}a\dot{D}O_2 = P_AO_2 - PaO_2$$

$$A\text{-}a\dot{D}O_2 = F_IO_2 (P_B - PH_2O) - \frac{PaCO_2}{R} - (PaO_2)$$

http://www.medicalc.com/frmls/pulmo/**AaDO2.htm**

age correction: 2.5 + 0.25(age)

↑ $Aa\dot{D}O_2$: diffusion defect, R → L shunt, $\dot{V}/Q$ mismatch.

Rule out R → L shunt: give 100% O_2 (10-15"), recalculate. diffusion and mild/moderate $\dot{V}/Q$ defects correct (at least partially).Shunts do not correct.

Diffusion defect ↑ $Aa\dot{D}O_2$ on 15% FIO_2, normal on 100%.

---

* RA= room air. R= right. L= left.
R = respiratory quotient (0.8).

SaO_2	Arterial O_2 saturation		**98%** (96-99%)
	Hb saturation:	PO_2 = 10.3	SO_2 = 10%
		PO_2 = 19.2	SO_2 = 30%
		PO_2 = 22.8	SO_2 = 40%
		PO_2 = **26.6**	SO_2 = **50%**
		PO_2 = 36.9	SO_2 = 70%
		PO_2 = 44.5	SO_2 = 80%
		PO_2 = 57.8	SO_2 = 90%
		PO_2 = 74.2	SO_2 = 95%
		PO_2 = 99.6	SO_2 = 97.5%
		PO_2 = 700	SO_2 = 99.95%
$S\bar{v}O_2$	Mixed Venous O_2 saturation		**70 - 80%**
P50	PaO_2 at which Hb is 50% saturated		**22 - 30 mmHg**

Hemoglobin Dissociation Curve

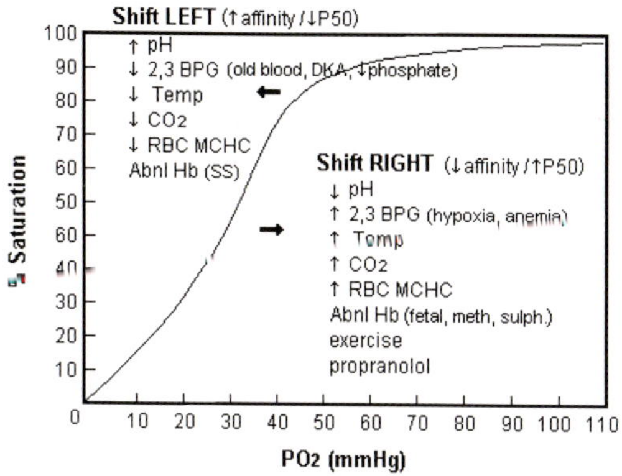

*Hb= hemoglobin. meth= methemoglobin. sulph= sulphemoglobin.
RBC= red blood cell. MCHC= mean corpuscular hemoglobin concentration.
DKA= diabetic ketoacidosis. 2, 3 BPG = 2, 3 biphosphoglycerate.

* SOURCE: Modified from *Medi*Formulas™, 1st ED (1998).

Gases

Oxygen Transport

RCFR	Red Cell Flow Rate RCFR= CI * Hct http://www.medicalc.com/frmls/pulmo/**RCFR.htm**	**1.2 L/min/m2**
OTRCM	O_2 Transport /Red Cell mass ratio OTRCM = $\dot{V}O_2$ / RCM http://www.medicalc.com/frmls/pulmo/**OTRCM.htm**	**0.12**
OTRCF	O_2 Transport /Red Cell Flow ratio OTRCF = $\dot{V}O_2$ / RCFR http://www.medicalc.com/frmls/pulmo/**OTRCF.htm**	**0.12**
TOEE	Tissue O_2 Extraction Efficiency TOEE = = $C(a-\bar{v})O_2$ / RCM http://www.medicalc.com/frmls/pulmo/**TOEE.htm**	**0.4**
TOEI	Tissue O_2 Extraction Index TOEI = = $C(a-\bar{v})O_2$ / RCFR http://www.medicalc.com/frmls/pulmo/**TOEI.htm**	**0.4**

Mechanics

FLOWS

FVC	Forced Vital Capacity (VC expired with maximum force)	$\geq$ **4.0 L**
FEVz	Forced Expiratory Volume (volume expired with maximum force in "z" seconds as a % of VC)	**FEV_1 = 83%** **FEV_2 = 94%** **FEV_3 = 97%**
$FEF_{25\text{-}75}$	Forced Mid-Expiratory Flow	**2.0 - 4.0 L/s**
$FIF_{25\text{-}75}$	Forced Inspiratory Flow	**5.0 L/s**
$FEF_{200\text{ - }1200}$	Forced Expiratory Flow	$\geq$ **3.5 L/s**

* VC = vital capacity.

Mechanics — PULMONARY

$FEF_{50\%}$	Forced Expiratory Flow at 50%	≥ **2.5 L/s**
$FEF_{75\%}$	Forced Expiratory Flow at 75%	≥ **1.5 L/s**
MVV	Maximal Voluntary Ventilation	**~170 L**

MVV = 40 * FEV_1 (F); 35 * FEV_1 (M).
MVV = VC * %air conductance

COMPLIANCE & PRESSURES

PEEP Positive End-Expiratory Pressure
(maximizes C_{stat} & minimizes QS/QT without ↓ C.O.).

MIF (NIF) Maximal Inspiratory Force **60- 100 cmH_2O**
(max pressure below atmospheric that a person can exert for 10-20" against a clossed glotis)
*also called NIF (negative inspiratory force).

MIP Maximal Inspiratory Pressure **60- 100 cmH_2O**

MEP Maximal Expiratory Pressure **~133 cmH_2O**

C_{stat} Static Compliance (ΔV/ΔP) **50-80 mL/cmH_2O**

$$C_{stat} = \frac{V_T}{(\text{Plateau Pressure} - \text{PEEP})}$$

http://www.medicalc.com/fmls/pulmo/**Cstat.htm**
If [illegible] 25-30 = "stiff lungs".

C_{stat} Static Compliance **100 mL/cmH_2O**
(lungs and thoracic cage)

C_{spec} Specific Compliance
C_{spec} = C_{stat} / FRC

*FRC = functional residual capacity. ΔV/ΔP = change in volume/change in pressure.

Mechanics

COMPLIANCE & PRESSURES (cont)

C_{dyn}	Dynamic Compliance $C_{dyn} = \frac{V_T}{(\text{Peak Pressure} - \text{PEEP})}$ http://www.medicalc.com/frmls/pulmo/**Cdyn.htm**	**50-80 mL/cmH_2O**
C_{dyn20}	Dynamic Compliance of 20 breaths/min	**0.25 L/cmH_2O**
P_{st} TLC	Static Recoil Pressure at TLC	**20 - 30 cmH_2O**

RESISTANCE & CONDUCTANCE

R_{aw}	Airway Resistance R_{aw} = Peak Pressure – Plateau Pressure 85 - 95% is from large airways.	
R_{aw}	Airway Resistance at FRC	**1.5 cmH_2O/L/s**
R_L	Pulmonary Resistance at FRC	**2.0 cmH_2O/L/s**
G_{aw}	Airway Conductance at FRC	**0.66 L/s/cmH_2O**
G_{aw}/V_L	Specific Conductance *0.22 per L of lung volume at which is measured.	**0.22***
W	Work of quiet Breathing	**0.5Kg*m/min**
W_{max}	Maximal Work of Breathing	**10Kg*m/breath**

* FRC = functional residual capacity. TLC = total lung capacity. VT = tidal volume.

Intubation / Extubation

INTUBATION CRITERIA*

- RR> 35-40/min
- $PaCO_2$ > 55mmHg (acute drop in blood pH).
- PaO_2 < 70 mmHg (on 100% O_2 mask)
- A–a Gradient > 400 (100% FIO_2)
- Bronchopulmonary toilet.
- Airway Protection.
- Inhalation injury (endoscopy/stridor).
- Head or spinal cord injury.
- ARDS

EXTUBATION CRITERIA*

- RR < 30/min
- $PaCO_2$ < 50 mmHg
- PaO_2 > 65mmHg (O_2 <40%)
- NIF < – 25 cm H_2O
- VT > 5mL/kg
- VC > 10mL/kg
- Resting MV < 10L/min
- ↑ consciousness (stable).
- Shunt < 20%
- VD/VT < 0.6

RR = respiratory rate.
NIF = negative inspiratory force.
VT = tidal volume.
VC = vital capacity.

* Individual Patient assessment required.

PFTs Patterns

CHANGES IN PULMONARY FUNCTION TESTS IN DISEASE STATES

Disease	Pulmonary Function Tests									
	VC/FVC	FEV	MVV	RV/FRC		FEF 25-75	TLC	MEF 50% VC	MIF 50% VC	DL
RESTRICTIVE LUNG DISEASE :										
Restrictive	↓	N/↑	N	↓	↓	↓	↓	N/↓	N	↓
OBSTRUCTIVE LUNG DISEASE :										
INTRATHORACIC:										
Emphysema	N/↓	↓	↓	↑	↑	↓	↑	↓	N	↓
Bronchitis	N/↓	↓	↓	↑	↑	↓	↑	↓	N	N
EXTRATHORACIC	N	↓	↓	N	N	↓	N	↓	↓	N
NeuroMuscular	N/↓	N	↓	N	N	N	N	N	N	N
Obesity	N/↓	N	N	N	↓	N	↓	N	N	N/↓

RENAL

Acid Base

AG Anion Gap **8 - 12 mEq/L**

$$AG = Na^+ - (Cl^- + HCO_3)$$

http://www.medicalc.com/frmls/renal/**AG.htm**

HCO3 deficit Bicarbonate deficit

$$HCO_3\ def = Wt\ (Kg) * 0.4 * (24 - HCO_3)$$

http://www.medicalc.com/frmls/renal/**HCO3_def.htm**

H+ def Acid deficit

$$H^+\ def = Wt\ (Kg) * 0.4 * (HCO_3 - 24)$$

http://www.medicalc.com/frmls/renal/**H_def.htm**

HCO3/PaCO2 ratio **1 : 2**

Henderson-Hasselbach equation

$$pH = 6.1 + \log \left\{ \frac{HCO_3}{(0.031 * PCO_2)} \right\}$$

Kassirer-Bleich equation H+ (nM/L)

$$H^+ = \frac{(24 * PaCO_2)}{HCO_3}$$

derived equations:

$$HCO_3 = \frac{(24 * PaCO_2)}{H^+}$$

$$PaCO_2 = \frac{(H^+ * HCO_3)}{24}$$

http://www.medicalc.com/frmls/renal/**KBE.htm**

*The Kassirer-Bleich equation is also called acid-base equation. Wt= weight.

Acid-Base Map

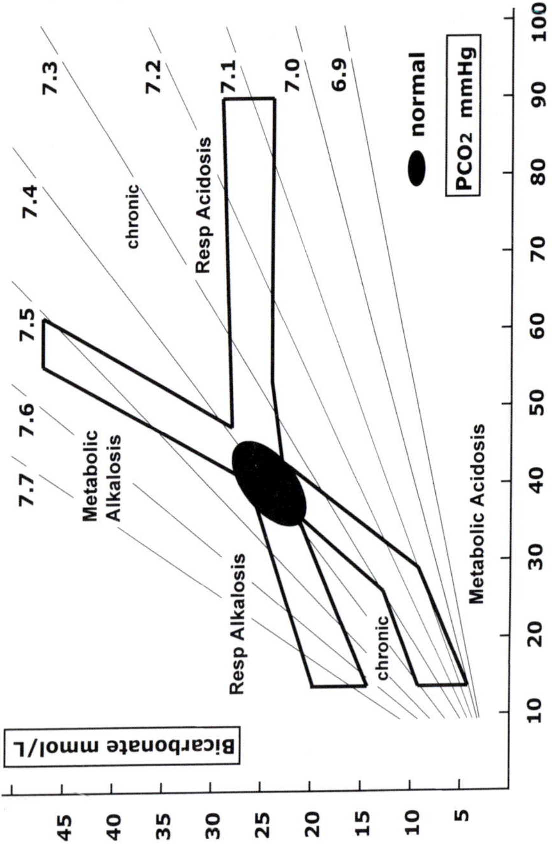

Acid - Base

[H+] in nEq/L from pH: nEq/L = nM/L

pH	[H+]	pH	[H+]	pH	[H+]	pH	[H+]
6.90	125						
6.92	120	7.12	76	7.32	48	7.52	30
6.94	115	7.14	73	7.34	46	7.54	29
6.96	110	7.16	70	7.36	44	7.56	28
6.98	105	7.18	66	7.38	42	7.58	27
7.00	100	7.20	63	**7.40**	**40**	7.60	25
7.02	95	7.22	60	7.42	38	7.62	24
7.04	91	7.24	58	7.44	37	7.64	23
7.06	87	7.26	55	7.46	35	7.66	22
7.08	83	7.28	52	7.48	33	7.68	21
7.10	80	7.30	50	7.50	32	7.70	20

Anion Gap

AG (S) Anion Gap (Serum) **8 - 16 mEq/L**

AG = Na^+ – (Cl^- + HCO_3)

http://www.medicalc.com/frmls/renal/**AG.htm**

<12 = diarrhea, RTA, $CaCl_2$, other acids

>15 = MUDPALES

(Methanol, Uremia, DKA, Paraldehyde, Alcoholic KA, Lactic acid, Ethylene glycol, Salicylates).

AG_4 Anion Gap (4 inputs) **12-16 mEq/L**

AG = (Na^+ + K^+) – (Cl^- + HCO_3)

http://www.medicalc.com/frmls/renal/**AG_4.htm**

*DKA = diabetic ketoacidosis. KA = ketoacidosis. RTA = renal tubular acidosis.

Anion Gap

AG (U) Anion Gap (Urine)**

$AG(U) = (Na^{+} + K^{+}) - Cl^{-}$

http://www.medicalc.com/frmls/renal/**AG_U.htm**

GI HCO_3 Loss		0		Renal HCO_3 Loss
– Gap	<————	|	————>	Gap +
+ NH_4	+		–	NH_4^+
(present)				(absent)

NH_4^+ Amonia (Urine)**, calculated

$NH_4^+ = Cl^{-} - (Na^{+} + K^{+}) + 80 mEq/L$

http://www.medicalc.com/frmls/renal/**NH4.htm**

**all values in Urine. GI = gastrointestinal

Acid-Base Compensations

pH	a: 7.38-7.44	(v: 7.36 ± 0.2)
PCO_2	a: 35-45 mmHg	(v: 46 ± 2)
PO_2	a: 80-100 mmHg	(v: 38± 5)
O_2 sat	a: > 97%	(v: 60- 80%)
HCO_3	a: 21-28 mmol/L	(v: 22-29)

Metabolic Acidosis ($\downarrow HCO_3 \rightarrow \downarrow PCO_2$)

PCO_2 $= 1.5(HCO_3) + 8 \pm 2$

PCO_2 = last 2 digits of pH

ΔPCO_2 = 1.0-1.3 mmHg ↓ for every 1 mmol/L ↓ in HCO_3

http://www.medicalc.com/frmls/renal/**MetAcid.htm**

Metabolic Alkalosis ($\uparrow HCO_3 \rightarrow \uparrow PCO_2$)

PCO_2 = variable change

PCO_2 $= 0.9(HCO_3) + 9$

ΔPCO_2 = 0.6-0.7 mmHg ↑ for every 1 mEq/L ↑ in HCO_3

http://www.medicalc.com/frmls/renal/**MetAlk.htm**

* a = arterial. v = venous.

Compensations RENAL

Respiratory Acidosis (↑PCO_2 → ↑HCO_3)

Acute

HCO_3 = 1.0 mmol/L ↑ for every 10 mmHg ↑ in PCO_2

Δ [H+] = 0.8 (Δ PCO_2)

http://www.medicalc.com/frmls/renal/**RespAcidA.htm**

Chronic

HCO_3 = 3.0-3.5 mmol/L ↑ for every 10 mmHg ↑ in PCO_2

Δ [H+] = 0.3 (Δ PCO_2)

http://www.medicalc.com/frmls/renal/**RespAcidC.htm**

Respiratory Alkalosis (↓PCO_2 → ↓HCO_3)

Acute

HCO_3 = 2.0-2.5 mmol/L ↓ for every 10 mmHg ↓ in PCO_2

Δ [H+] = 0.8 (Δ PCO_2)

http://www.medicalc.com/frmls/renal/**RespAlkA.htm**

Chronic

HCO_3 = 4.0-5.0 mmol/L ↓ for every 10 mmHg ↓ in PCO_2

Δ [H+] = 0.17 (Δ PCO_2)

http://www.medicalc.com/frmls/renal/**RespAlkC.htm**

Renal Tubular Acidosis

	Proximal	**Classical Distal**	**Type 4**	**↑ K+ Distal**
Prevalence	Rare	Rare	↑ Common	Common
K+ (plasma)	Low	Low	High	High
pH (urine)	< 6	> 6	< 6	variable
NH_4^+ (urine)	normal	Low	Low	Low
Defect	↓ high cap. HCO_3 transp.	↓ H+ pump	↓ NH_3 gen. ↓ aldo effect	↓ Distal Na+ transport
Rx	Diuretic	HCO_3	Diuretic	HCO_3
cause e.g.	acetazolamide	amphotericin	Diabetes	Obstruction

*aldo = aldosterone. cap = capacity. gen = generation.

Acidosis

Elevated Anion Gap Acidoses

	Acid	AG	Osm Gap	Findings Chemical	Clinical
Renal failure "uremic"	PO_4 SO_4 organic	15-25	N	BUN > 40 Cr > 4 PO_4 > 6	Hx of renal disease
Ketosis	AcAc, BHB	>20	N		
diabetes				↑ glucose	diabetes
etOH				false ↑ cr	Alcoholism
Toxins					
ethylene glycol	glycocolic others	>20	↑ >10	Ca oxalate crystalluria	renal, cns cardiac
methanol	formic others	>20	↑	↑ amylase	retinal edema papillitis
paraldehyde	unknown	>20	N	ketones	paraldehyde odor
salycilates	mixed organic	15-20	N	assoc resp alk.	+ children

* AcAc = acetoacetate. BHB= beta-hydroxy-butyrate. cr= creatinine.

Acidosis and Alcohol ingestion *

	organ	Osm Gap	ketone bodies	Breath	Acidosis
ethanol	liver	↑	±	+++	0
methanol	eyes	↑	0	—	+++
ethylene glycol	kidney	↑	0	—	+++
isopropyl		↑	±	+	0
etoh KA		N	±	+	+

(ethylene glycol: urine shows oxalate hippurate crystals).

Tx for methanol/ethylene glycol intox: give ethanol/hemodialysis

* see also osmolality. * KA= ketoAcidosis.

Clearances RENAL

ClCr Creatinine Clearance **91-130 mL/min**

$$Cl\ Cr = \frac{Cr,\ mg/mL\ (U) * Urine\ Vol\ (mL/min)}{Cr,\ mg/mL\ (S)}$$

* Result x 100.

http://www.medicalc.com/frmls/renal/**Clcr.htm**

$$Cl\ Cr = \frac{Cr,\ mg/day\ (U)}{Cr,\ mg/mL\ (S)} \times 70$$

GFR Glomerular filtration rate, estimated mL/min

$$GFR = \frac{(140 - age) * weight\ (Kg)}{72 * Cr\ (S)}$$

http://www.medicalc.com/frmls/renal/**GFR.htm**

*Female value = multiply result by 0.85

* GFR assesses glomerular filtration primarily.

Normal Values = F : 85-105 mL/min*
M : 100-130 mL/min*

Cl Urea Urea Clearance **64 - 99 mL/min**

$$Cl\ urea = \frac{UUN\ (mg/mL) * Urine\ Vol\ (mL/min)}{BUN\ (mg/mL)}$$

*glomerular filtration and partial tubular reabsorption.

http://www.medicalc.com/frmls/renal/**Clurea.htm**

Cl PAH p-Aminohippurate Clearance mL/min

*effective renal plasma flow and tubular function.

F : 594±102 mL/min M : 654±163 mL/min

Cl H_2O Free Water Clearance **25 - 100 mL/h**

Cl H_2O = Urinary Output – Cl osm

http://www.medicalc.com/frmls/renal/**ClH2O.htm**

Cl Osm Osmolar Clearance **120 mL/h**

Cl Osm = (U osm/P osm) x Urine Output

http://www.medicalc.com/frmls/renal/**Closm.htm**

Phenolsulfonphtalein (IV dose) > 25% in 15 min*

*assesses mainly tubular secretion. 60-80% in 2 hours

---

*Normal values corrected to 1.73m2 BSA. Cl = clearance. M= male. F= female. S= serum. U= urine. Vol= volume. Osm= osmolality.

Oliguria

DIAGNOSTIC INDICES IN RENAL FAILURE

Variable (units)	prerenal	renal
FENa+ (%)	< 1%	> 1%
FE Urea (%)	< 20-30%	> 40-70%
RFI (%) *	< 1%	> 1%
BUN / Cr (S) (ratio)	> 20	< 10-15
Cr(U)/**Cr**(S) (ratio)	> 40	< 20
UUN/BUN (ratio)	> 8	< 3
Osm(U)/**Osm**(S) (ratio)	> 1.3	< 1.1
Na+ (U) (mmol/L)	< 10	> 20
Osm (U) (mOsm/Kg)	> 500	< 250
Sp Gr (U)	> 1.018	< 1.012
Urine Sediment	hyaline casts	muddy brown granular casts

S= serum. U= urine. Vol= volume. Osm= osmolality.

Prerenal: ECF volume depletion, CHF, ↓ BP,

Renal: ATN (75% of all cases), postop, contrast, ABO, toxins, all prerenal causes that release pigment (transfusion, rhabdo, crush), eclampsia, sepsis, acute interstitial nephritis, AGN, malignant HTN, vasculitis, uric acid nephropathy, ↑Ca++, HUS, hepatorenal syndrome.

PostRenal: bilateral ureteral / bladder outlet obstruction.

RFI Renal Failure Index

$$RFI = \frac{Na+ (U)}{Cr (U) / Cr (S)}$$

http://www.medicalc.com/frmls/renal/**RFI.htm**

* FENa & FE urea, see fractional excretions.

Fractional Excretions RENAL

FENa+ FE of Sodium * < 1% (normal, prerenal)

$$\text{FE Na+ (\%)} = \frac{\text{Na+ (U, mmol/L)} * \text{Cr (S, mg/mL)}}{\text{Na+ (S, mmol/L)} * \text{Cr (U, mg/mL)}}$$

* Result x 100. * % of filtered Na+ load excreted.

http://www.medicalc.com/frmls/renal/**FENa.htm**

FE Urea FE of Urea * < 35% (prerenal)

$$\text{FE Urea (\%)} = \frac{\text{Urea (U, g/d)} * \text{Cr (S, mg/dL)}}{\text{BUN (mg/dL)} * \text{Cr (U, g/d)}}$$

* Result x 100. * not altered by diuretics

http://www.medicalc.com/frmls/renal/**FEUrea.htm**

FE Uric a FE of Uric acid * < 10% (prerenal)

$$\text{FE Urica (\%)} = \frac{\text{Uric (U, mg/dL)} * \text{Cr (S, mg/dL)}}{\text{Uric (S, mg/dL)} * \text{Cr (U, mg/dL)}}$$

* Result x 100.

http://www.medicalc.com/frmls/renal/**FEUrica.htm**

TTKG

TTKG Transtubular Potassium Gradient

$$\text{TTKG} = \frac{\text{K+ (U, mmol/L)} * \text{Osm (S, mOsm/Kg)}}{\text{K+ (S, mmol/L)} * \text{Osm (U, mOsm/Kg)}}$$

http://www.medicalc.com/frmls/renal/**TTKG.htm**

Nl values: 4% - 14% (varies with diet).

Hypokalemia :
- < 2 = GI loss
- > 4 = renal loss (excess aldo)

Hyperkalemia:
- < 6 = renal (↓ aldo)
- >10= non-renal (nl aldo effect)

* The FENa formula presented here is equivalent to FENa = (Na U/P)/(Cr U/P). The same is true for the other formulas repectively. P = plasma. S = serum. U = urine.

Amylase/Creatinine Cl ratio

AmCr_Cl Amylase/Creatinine Clearance ratio

$$AmCr\_Cl = \frac{\text{amylase (U)} * \text{Cr (S, mg/mL)}}{\text{amylase (S)} * \text{Cr (U, mg/mL)}}$$

* Result x 100. Urine values from spot urine.

http://www.medicalc.com/frmls/renal/**AmCr_Cl.htm**

< 1% and hyperamylasemia = suggests macroamylasemia.

> 5% = acute pancreatitis

Sodium

Na+ def Sodium Deficit **0 mmol**

Na+ def = 0.6(Wt)(140 – Na+) **+** (140)(volume def, L)

* Wt in Kg.

http://www.medicalc.com/frmls/renal/**Na_def.htm**

Na+ correction (glucose)

Δ Na+ = ((0.016) * (glucose – 100))

Na+_corr = measured Na+ **+** ((0.016)*(glucose – 100))

Na+ (S) ↓ 1.35 mEq/L per 100mg% ↑ glucose
↓ 0.3-0.4mEq/L per mmol/L ↑ glucose

http://www.medicalc.com/frmls/renal/**Na_corr.htm**

(Na+ in mmol/L. Glucose in mg/dL.).

FENa+ see fractional excretions

Chloride

Cl- def Chloride Deficit **0 mmol**

Cl- def = 0.5(Wt) (103 – measured Cl-)

http://www.medicalc.com/frmls/renal/**Cl_def.htm**

* Wt in Kg. Cl-= mEq/L

*Notice that in these Sodium and Chloride formulas, measured Na must be ≥ 140, glucose ≥ 100 and Chloride ≥ 103 (to prevent results from being negative).

Water

RENAL

TBW Total Body Water **~60% of BW**

TBW, L = 0.6 * Wt (Kg)

http://www.medicalc.com/frmls/renal/**TBW.htm**

TBS Total Body Solute

TBS = TBW (L) * Osmolality

http://www.medicalc.com/frmls/renal/**TBS.htm**

H2O_xs Free Water excess **0 L**

H2O_xs = TBW * {1– [Na+/140]}

http://www.medicalc.com/frmls/renal/**H2O_xs.htm**

H2O gain

$$H_2O \text{ gain} = 0.6 * wt - \left(0.6 * wt * \frac{osm}{290} \right)$$

* Wt in Kg.

http://www.medicalc.com/frmls/renal/**H2Ogain.htm**

H2O load (20mL/Kg) nl= 80% excreted in 4h
U osm < 100

Lactate excess

L_xs Lactate excess **0**

$$L\_xs = (L_{PT} - L_{NL}) - (P_{PT} - P_{NL}) + \frac{L_{NL}}{P_{NL}}$$

LPT= patient lactate. LNL= normal Lactate: 1.0mmol/L.
PPT= patient pyruvate. PNL normal pyruvate: 0.1mmol/L.

http://www.medicalc.com/frmls/renal/**L_xs.htm**

Uric acid

UaCr_r Uric acid / creatinine ratio **< 1.0**

$$UaCr\_r = \frac{\text{spot urine Uric acid}}{\text{spot urine Creatinine}}$$

*in mg/dL.

http://www.medicalc.com/frmls/renal/**UaCr_r.htm**

> 1.0 = suspect acute uric acid nephropathy.

*normal lactate/pyruvate ratio = 10:1.

Potassium

K+ Total Body Potassium **55 mEq/Kg**

K+ = 0.55 * Wt (Kg)

http://www.medicalc.com/frmls/renal/**TBK.htm**

K+ def Potassium Deficit, Body **0 mmol**

K+ def = ~370mEq for each mEq/L fall in serum.

FEK+ Fractional Excretion of K+* **%**

$$\text{FE K+} = \frac{\text{K+ (U, mmol/L)} * \text{Cr (S, mg/mL)}}{\text{K+ (S, mmol/L)} * \text{Cr (U, mg/mL)}}$$

* Result x 100, in % terms.

http://www.medicalc.com/frmls/renal/**FEK.htm**

K+ correction (pH) K+ ↑ 0.6 mEq/L per 0.1 ↓ pH

K+ correction (Osm) K+ ↑ 0.6 mEq/L per 10 mOsm ↑ (serum)

K+ correction (pH) K+ ↑ 0.15 mEq/L per 100x10^9 platelets/L

* all K+ in mmol/L in serum. Osm = serum Osmolality. pH in blood.

Calcium

Ca_pb protein-bound Calcium **50-54% of total**

pb_Ca = (albumin * 8) + (globulin * 2) + 3

http://www.medicalc.com/frmls/endo/**Ca_pb.htm**

Ca++ correction (albumin) **/CaAlb_c.htm**

Ca++_corr = Ca++ **+** ((1.0)*(4.0 – albumin))

Ca++ (P) ↓ 0.8mg% per each g% ↓ albumin

Ca++ correction (globulin) **/CaGlob_c.htm**

Ca++_corr = Ca++ **+** ((0.16)*(globulin – 3.5))

Ca++ (P) ↓ 0.16mg% per each g% ↑ globulin

Ca++ correction (pH) **/CapH_c.htm**

$$\text{Ca++\_corr} = \text{Ca++} + \left(0.12 * \frac{(\text{pH} - 7.4)}{0.1} \right)$$

Ca++ (P) ↓ 0.12mg% per each 0.1 ↑ pH units

* Ca++ (serum, mg/dL). Albumin and Globulin (serum, g/dL).

*corr = corrected.

Phosphate RENAL

FEPi Fractional Excretion of Pi* **10 - 20%**

$$FE\ Pi = \frac{PO_4\ (U,\ mmol/L) * Cr\ (S,\ mg/mL)}{PO_4\ (S,\ mmol/L) * Cr\ (U,\ mg/mL)}$$

* Result x 100, in % terms.

http://www.medicalc.com/frmls/renal/**FEPi.htm**

TRP Tubular Reabsorption of Phosphate **82 - 95%**

TRP = 1 – (FEPi / 100)

* Result x 100, in % terms.

http://www.medicalc.com/frmls/renal/**TRP.htm**

Phosphate Therapy

ORAL 250 - 500mg PO QID *always oral if PO4 >2mg/dL

K-Phos tab = 250mg PO4 (8mM) & 1.4 mEq K+ & 13.1mEq Na+

Neutra-Phos tab = 250mg PO4 (8mM) & 7.1 mEq K+ & 7.1mEq Na+

Fleets-Phosphosoda=128mg PO4/mL(4mM/mL) & 4.8mEq Na+(5mL)

IV			
	uncomplicated	0.08 - 0.2 mM/Kg	over 6 hours
	prolonged	0.16 - 0.24 mM/Kg	

Na-Phos (15mL/amp) = 3mM/mL PO4 & 4.0 mEq/mL Na+

K-Phos (15mL/amp) = 3mM/mL PO4 & 4.4 mEq/mL K+

Osmolality

Osm Osmolality (Serum) **285-295mOsmol/Kg**

$$Osm = 2(Na^{+} + K^{+}) + \frac{glucose}{18} + \frac{Urea}{2.8} + \frac{etOH}{4.6}$$

http://www.medicalc.com/frmls/renal/**OsmS.htm**

Osmolar Gap **< 10 mOsmol/Kg**

Osm Gap = measured Osm – calculated Osm

http://www.medicalc.com/frmls/renal/**OsmG.htm**

states:
1.- calc > measured = lab error, arithmetical error.
2.- measured Osm nl, calc Osm low = ↓water (S)
3.- measured Osm ↑↑, calc Osm ↑ or nl = presence of unmeasured osmol (+ osmolar gap)

Substance	Mol weight	Osmolal Gap (at that level)
Ethanol	46	80 mOsm/Kg H_2O
Ethyl ether	26	70
Isopropanol	60	60
Methanol	32	27
Acetone	58	10
Ethylene glycol	62	4

Differential Diagnosis algorithm

↑ Osm -->	nl pH -->	no acetone -->	ethanol
		acetone -->	isopropanol
	↓ pH -->	-->	methanol
		-->	ethylene glycol

*etOH= ethanol. nl = normal. osm = osmolality.

BODY FLUIDS

Composition

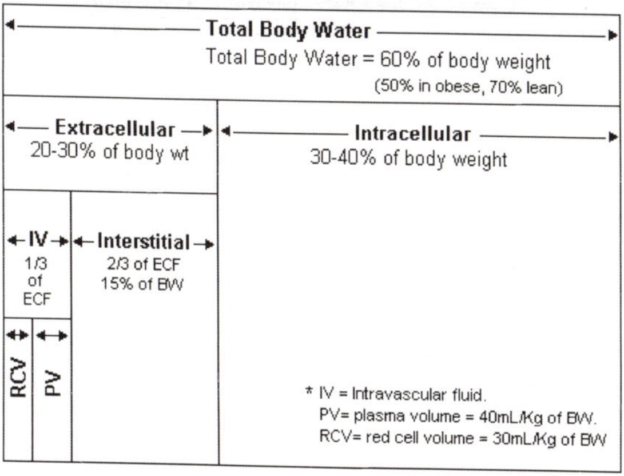

Electrolyte Composition

	Plasma	Interstitial	Intracellular
CATIONS	Na+ 142 K+ 4 Ca++ 5 Mg++ 2 total = 153	Na+ 145 K+ 4 total = 149	Na+ ~10 K+ 156 Ca++ 3.3 Mg++ 26 total = 195.3
ANIONS	Cl- 104 HCO3- 27 HPO4 2 SO4 1 org acids 6 protein 13 total = 153	Cl- 114 HCO3- 31 total = 145	Cl- 2 HCO3- 8 HPO4 95 SO4 20 protein 55 total = 180

Miscellaneos Fluids

FLUIDS * d = day. L = liter.

(mEq/L)	Na+	K+	Cl-	HCO3-	Volume/d
Bile	145	5	95	35-50	1.5L
Gastric	80	10	100		2.0L
diarrhea	40	50	30	30-45	
ileostomy	125	10	55	50-70	0.5-2L
jejunum	100	5	100	10	—
pancreatic	140	5	65	70-90	0.7-1L
saliva	60	20	15	50	1.0L
sweat	50	5	40	—	0.1 - 4.0L

IV SOLUTIONS

SALTS & SOLUTIONS (conversions)

Salt Name	Salt Formula	mEq per mg of salt	mg of salt per mEq
Sodium chloride	$NaCl$	17.1*	58.4
sodium bicarbonate	$NaHCO_3$	11.9	84
sodium sulfate	$NaSO_4 \cdot 10H_2O$	6	161
potassium chloride	KCl	13.4	74.6
Potassium bicarb	$KHCO_3$	10	100
calcium carbonate	$CaCO_3$	10	100
calcium chloride	$CaCl_2 \cdot 2H_2O$	14	73
calcium gluconate	$Ca\text{-}gluc_2 \cdot 1H_2O$	4	224
calcium lactate	$Ca\text{-}lact_2 \cdot 5H_2O$	6	154
magnesium sulfate	$MgSO_4 \cdot 7H_2O$	8	123
ammonium chloride	NH_4Cl	18.7	53.5

* 1g Na+ = 43mEq (4g Na+ = 10g NaCl, approximately).

IV Solutions

IV SOLUTIONS

	(mEq/L)				Dextrose		
	Na+	K+	Cl-	HCO3- (base)	mOsm/L	g/L	kcal/L
5% D/W					278	50	170
10% D/W					556	100	340
20% D/W					1112	200	680
50% D/W					2780	500	1700
70% D/W					3892	700	2380
0.45%NaCl	77		77		154		0
0.85%NaCl	145		145		290		0
0.9%NaCl	154		154		308		0
3% NaCl	513		513		1026		
5%NaCl	855		855		1710		
D5½NS	77		77		421	50	170
D5NS	154		154		564	50	170
RL	130	4	109	28 lactate	272	0	0
D5RL	130	4	109	28 lactate	550	50	170
5%albumin	145		145		290		
25%albumin	145		145		290		
dextran40	154		154		310		
dextran70	154		154		010		

*D/W = dextrose in water (1g dextrose provides 3.4 kcal). NS= normal saline.

Albumin

5% ——>	50mL	=	2.5 g
	100mL	=	5.0 g
	250mL	=	12.5 g
	500mL	=	25.0 g
10% ——>	20mL	=	2.0 g
	25mL	=	2.5 g
	50mL	=	5.0 g
	100mL	=	10.0 g

Parenteral Additives

PARENTERAL ADDITIVES

Additive	Concentration	vol/amp (mL)	mEq/amp
7.5% sodium bicarbonate	0.9mEq/mL	50	46.6
42% sodium phosphate*	3.0mmol/mL PO4	15	45 P
7.5% potassium chloride	1.0mEq/mL K+	20	20
15% potassium chloride**	2.0mEq/mL K+	30	60
46% potassium phosphate*	3.0mmol/mL PO4	15	45 P
10% calcium chloride		10	13.6
10% calcium gluconate		10	4.6
50% magnesium sulfate		10	40.6
27% ammonium chloride		20	100
50% glucose	500mg/mL	50	25g
25% mannitol	250mg/mL	50	12.5g

* also contains 4.0mEq/mL Na+. ** also contains 45mM PO4.

IV Infusions

IV INFUSIONS

1mL = 20 drops = 60 microdrops.

1 **Dopamine** 400mg/500mL =
0.8mg/mL = 800ug/mL = 800ug/60microdrops
13.33ug/microdrop

2 **Dosage = ug/kg/min** (e.g) = 5ug/70Kg/min = 350ug/min

3 **Total dose/min (TDM)** = 350ug/min

4 **dose in microdrops/min =** $\frac{\text{TDM}}{\text{[microdrop]}} = \frac{\text{350ug/min}}{\text{13.33ug/microdrop}}$

= 26.2 microdrops/min

Dopamine 800mg/500mL = 26.66ug/microdrop.
Dobutamine 250mg/500mL = 8.33ug/microdrop.
Dobutamine 500mg/500mL = 16.66ug/microdrop.

*calculate with drops when using regular tubing, microdrops when using microtubing.

DRUGS

Adenosine (Adenocard):
IVP: 6mg (1 - 3 sec) then 12mg

Aminocaproic acid (Amicar):
Diluent: D5W or NS. Conc: 4–5g/250mL.
IV: 4–5g over 1h, then 1.0–1.25g/h

Aminophylline:
Diluent: NS or D5W. Conc: 1000mg/500mL = 2mg/mL
IV loading dose:6mg/kg over 6h
IV Infusion (non-smokers): 0.3–0.5mg/kg/h
IV Infusion (smokers): 0.7 – 0.9mg/kg/h

Amrinone (Inocor):
Diluent: NS only. Conc: 500mg/500mL = 1mg/mL
IV: 0.75mg/kg (over 2 - 3 min) then,
IV Infusion: 5.0–15.0ug/kg/min

Atenolol:
IV: 5–10mg over 5 min.

Atropine SO_4:
IVP: 1.0mg (asystole, total 3mg)
IVP: 0.5–1.0mg (bradycardia, total 3mg)

Bicarbonate, Sodium:
IVP: 1.0mEq/kg then 0.5mEq/kg q10min

Bretylium Tosylate:
Diluent: D5W or NS. Conc: 2g/500mL = 4mg/mL
IVP: 5.0mg/kg in 1 min (total: 30-35mg/kg)
IV Infusion: 1.0–2.0mg/min (2g/500mL D5W)

Bumetanide (Bumex):
IV or IM: 0.5–1.0mg over 1–2min

Calcium chloride (10%):
IV: 2.0 – 4.0mg/kg q10min (as needed)

Digoxin:
IV/PO loading: 10–15ug/kg over 12–24hours
(0.5mg IV over 5min --> 0.25mg q6h x2–4)

Diazepam (Valium):
IV: 2–10mg (not to exceed 5mg/min)

* IM= intramuscular. IV= intravenous. IVP= IV push. PO= oral. SL= sublingual. D5W = dextrose 5% in water. NS = normal saline. Conc = concentration.

Drugs

Diltiazem (Cardizem):

Diluent: D5W or NS. Conc: 250mg/500mL = 0.5mg/mL
IV: 20mg or 0.25mg/kg (then 0.35mg/kg)
IV Infusion: 5 – 15mg/h

Diphenhydramine (Benadryl):

Dose: 10–50mg (slow IV, or deep IM, PO)

Dobutamine (Dobutrex):

Diluent: D5W or NS. Conc: 250mg/500mL = 0.5mg/mL
IV: 2 – 20ug/kg/min

Dopamine (Intropin):

Diluent: D5W or NS. Conc: 800mg/500mL 1600ug/mL
dopaminergic: 1 – 3ug/kg/min IV
β-adrenergic: 3 – 10ug/kg/min IV
α-adrenergic: > 10ug/kg/min IV

Epinephrine: (1:1000)

Diluent: NS. Conc: 1mg/250mL = 4ug/mL
IVP: 1.0 mg q3–5min (then 5mg or 0.1mg/kg)
IV Infusion: 2 – 10ug/min

Esmolol: (2.5g/250mL D5W or NS = 10mg/mL)

IVP: 500ug/kg over 1 min
IV Infusion: start at 50ug/kg/min

Flumazenil (Mazicon):

IV: 0.2mg over 30 sec (max 3.0mg/h)

Furosemide (Lasix):

IV: 20–80mg over 1–2min

Heparin:

Diluent: D5W or NS.
Concentration: 25,000 units/500mL = 50u/mL
IV Bolus: 5,000 units X 1
IV Infusion: 1000–1300 units/h

Insulin:

Diluent: NS. Conc: 100units/250mL = 0.4 units/mL
IVP: 0.1 units/kg

Ipecac:

PO: 30mL (follow with 1–2 glasses of water)

* IM= intramuscular. IV= intravenous. IVP= IV push. PO= oral. SL= sublingual. D5W = dextrose 5% in water. NS = normal saline. Conc = concentration.

DRUGS

Isoproterenol (Isuprel):

Diluent: D5W or NS. Conc: 1mg/250mL = 4ug/mL
IV Infusion: 2 – 10ug/min

Labetalol (Normodyne):

Diluent: D5W, NS, RL. Conc: 200mg/200mL = 1mg/mL
IV: 20mg over 2min, -->40–80mg (max 300mg)
IV Infusion: 2mg/min

Lidocaine:

Diluent: D5W or NS. Conc: 2g/500mL = 4mg/mL
IVP: 1.0 – 1.5mg/kg (x2 q5–10min)
IV Infusion: 2 – 4mg/min

Lorazepam:

IV or deep IM: 2–4mg (not to exceed 2mg/min)

Magnesium:

IV Infusion: 1 – 2g/100mL D5W (2min)

Mannitol (20%):

IV: 1.5 – 2.0g/kg over 30–60min

Metoprolol:

IV: 5mg q5min x 3 (slow push)

Morphine SO_4:

IV: 1 – 3mg q5min (until desired response)

Naloxone (Narcan):

IV: 0.4 – 2.0mg q2min prn (up to 10mg)

Nicardipine:

Diluent: D5W or NS. Conc: 25mg/250mL = 0.1mg/mL
IV Infusion: 2.0mg/h

Nifedipine (Procardia):

SL: 10mg (have Patient chew and swallow)

Nitroglycerin:

Diluent: D5W or NS. Conc: 50mg/250mL = 200ug/mL
IV Infusion: 10 – 300ug/min

Nitroprusside Na+ (Nitropress):

Diluent: D5W only. Conc: 100mg/500mL = 200ug/mL
IV Infusion: 0.1 – 5.0ug/kg/min

---

* IM= intramuscular. IV= intravenous. IVP= IV push. PO= oral. SL= sublingual. D5W = dextrose 5% in water. NS = normal saline. Conc = concentration.

Drugs

Norepinephrine (Levophed):

Diluent: D5W only. Conc: 4mg/250mL = 16ug/mL
IV Infusion: 0.5 – 1.0ug/min (up to 30ug/min)

Pancuronium (Pavulon):

IV: 0.06 – 0.10mg/kg

Phenytoin (Dilantin):

IV: 10 – 15mg/kg (not to exceed 50mg/min)

Phenylephrine (Neo-synephrine):

Diluent: D5W or NS. Conc: 10mg/250mL = 0.04mg/mL
IV Infusion: 0.04mg/min

Procainamide (Pronestyl):

Diluent: D5W. Conc: 1g/250mL = 4mg/mL
IV Infusion: 20mg/min (total: 17mg/kg)
IV maintenance Infusion: 1 – 4mg/min

Streptokinase:

IV: 1.5million units over 1h

Succinylcholine (Anectine):

IV Infusion: 0.6mg/kg over 10–30sec (max = 150mg)

TPA (Alteplase, Activase):

IV: 100mg (15mg bolus, then 50mg in 1h, then 35mg in 1h)

Vercuronium (Norcuron):

IV: 0.08–0.1mg/kg

Verapamil:

IV: 2.5–5.0mg over 2 min (x4 q15–30min)

---

* IM= intramuscular. IV= intravenous. IVP= IV push. PO= oral. SL= sublingual. D5W = dextrose 5% in water. NS = normal saline. Conc = concentration.

IMPORTANT NOTICE:
The package insert for each drug should be consulted routinely for use and dosage prior to prescription and/or administration.

Heparin

IV Heparin Standard Schedule*:

Initial dose:	5000u (bolus) --> 1000u/h
APTT < 35s	5000u (bolus) --> ↑ rate 200u/h
APTT 35s–45s	2500u (bolus) --> ↑ rate 100u/h
APTT 46s–70s	no change
APTT 71s–90s	↓ infusion by 100u/h
APTT > 90s	hold infusion for 1h, then ↓ rate by 200u/h

(Heparin= 25,000 units/500mL D5W)
APTT = activated partial thromboplastin time
*Individual Patient adjustment required.

Insulin Sliding Scale

INSULIN SLIDING SCALE *:

blood glucose level (mg/dL):	regular Insulin dose (U):
> 400	call MD
351–400	10 – 12
301–350	8 – 10
251–300	6 – 8
201–250	4 – 6
151–200	2 – 4
75–150	do nothing
< 75	call MD

*Individual Patient adjustment required.

* ↑ = increrase. ↓ = decrease. u/h = units per hour.

OVERDOSAGE

SUBSTANCE/POISON	ANTIDOTE	DOSAGE for ADULTS
Acetaminophen	N-acetylcysteine	140mg/kg PO, followed by 70mg/kg q4h x 17doses
Anticholinergics	Physostigmine sulfate	0.5–2.0mg IV (IM) over 2 min q30-60min prn
Anticholinesterases	Atropine sulfate	1.5mg IV (IM SC) q15min prn (dry secretions).
	Pralidoxime*	1g IV (PO) over 15–30min q8–12h x 3doses prn
Carbon monoxide	Oxygen	100% hyperbaric
Cyanide	Amyl nitrite	inhalation pearls for 15–30sec q1min
	Sodium Nitrate	followed by Sodium Nitrate 300mg IV over 3min, , repeated in half dosage in 2h prn
	Sodium Thiosulfate	followed by Na+ Thiosulfate, 12.5g IV over 10min , repeated in half dosage in 2h prn
Digoxin	AntiDigoxin Fab fragments	Acute ingestion: dose (vials) = [ingested digoxin (mg) **x** 0.8] / 0.6 Chronic ingestion: dose (vials) = [level (S, ng/mL) **x** Wt (kg)] / 100, infused in 0.9%saline over 15–30min, repeat prn.

THIS IS ONLY A GUIDE, ANTIDOTE USAGE AN DOSE WILL DEPEND ON THE SPECIFIC CLINICAL SITUATION, CONTACT THE POISON CONTROL CENTER FOR SPECIFIC THERAPEUTIC RECOMMENDATIONS.

*Pralidoxime is indicated in organophosphate poisoning.

SUBSTANCE/POISON	ANTIDOTE	DOSAGE for ADULTS
Ethylene glycol	ethano	0.6g/kg of ethanol in 5% D/W IV (PO) over 30–45 min, followed by 110mg/kg/h (to maintain a blood alcohol level of 100–150mg/dL.
Heavy metals (arsenic, copper, gold, mercury)	Chelators:	
	EDTA	1.0g IV (IM) in NS over 1h q12h
	Dimercaprol (BAL)	2.5–5.0 mg/kg IM q4–6h
	Penicillamine	250–500 mg PO q6h
	DMSA	10mg/kg PO tid x 5days then bid x 14days
Iron	deferoxamine	I.0g IM (IV at <15mg/kg/h if hypotension) q8h prn
Isoniazid (INH)	Pyridoxine	amount = estimated INH ingestion, up to 5g over 30–60min
Methanol	ethanol	see ehtylene glycol
Methemoglobimemia	methylene blue	1–2mg/kg IV over 5 min, repeat in 1h prn
Opioids	Naloxone hydrochloride	0.4–2.0mg IV (IM, SC, endotracheally) prn
Warfarin and related drugs	Vitamin K (phytonadione)	10mg IM, SC, or IV (if IV, over 20min)
	Fresh-frozen plasma	as needed.

THIS IS ONLY A GUDE, ANTIDOTE USAGE AN DOSE WILL DEPEND ON THE SPECIFIC CLINICAL SITUATION, CONTACT THE POISON CONTROL CENTER FOR SPECIFIC THERAPEUTIC RECOMMENDATIONS.

NUTRITION

BSA Body Surface Area **1.7m²**

$$BSA = Wt^{0.425}(kg) \times Ht^{0.725}(cm) \times .007184$$

* normal values for an 170 cm-height, 70-kg adult male.

http://www.medicalc.com/frmls/nutrition/**BSA.htm**

IBW Ideal Body Weight

$$IBW\ (M) = Ht^2\ (m) \times 23$$

$$IBW\ (F) = Ht^2\ (m) \times 21.5$$

http://www.medicalc.com/frmls/nutrition/**IBW.htm**

IBW hamwi method

M = 106Lb for the first 5 ft + 6Lb for each additional inch.
M = 48kg for the first 152.4cm + 1.1kg for each additional cm
F = 100Lb for the first 5 ft + 5Lb for each additional inch
F = 45kg for the first 152.4cm + 0.9kg for each additional cm

http://www.medicalc.com/frmls/nutrition/**IBWhamwi.htm**

ABW Adjusted Body Weight * **kg**

ABW = IBW + [(actual BW – IBW) * 0.25]

* calculated only if actual BW is more than 125% of IBW

http://www.medicalc.com/frmls/nutrition/**ABW.htm**

%IBW percentage of Ideal Body Weight **%**

%IBW = (actual Wt * 100) / IBW

http://www.medicalc.com/frmls/nutrition/**IBWpc.htm**

* Wt and IBW in Kg (or both in lb).

BMI Body Mass Index **23–27kg/m2**

$$BMI = \frac{wt\ (kg)}{ht^2\ (m)}$$

http://www.medicalc.com/frmls/nutrition/**BMI.htm**

---

*formulas for adults.

Metabolism

BMR Basal Metabolic Rate **kcal/m2/h**

BMR = 37 – [(age (y) – 20)/10]

http://www.medicalc.com/frmls/nutrition/**BMR.htm**

HBE Harris-Benedict Equation: Basal Energy Expenditure **kcal/d**

M = 66 + (13.7*Wt, kg) + (5*Ht, cm) – (6.8*age, y)

F = 655 + (9.6*Wt, kg) + (1.8*Ht, cm) – (4.7*age, y)

http://www.medicalc.com/frmls/nutrition/**HBE.htm**

EE Energy Expenditure

EE = CO * Hb * ((SaO_2 - SvO_2)/100) * 95

http://www.medicalc.com/frmls/nutrition/**EE.htm**

* CO= cardiac output (L/min).
* Hb = hemoglobin (g/dL).
* SaO2 and SvO2 = arterial and venous O2 saturations (%).

BEE Basal Energy Expenditure (easy-estimate)

BEE = 25 – 30 kcal/kg

http://www.medicalc.com/frmls/nutrition/**BEE.htm**

TEE Total Energy Expenditure **kcal**

TEE = BEE * AF * SF

AF: activity factor. Bed rest= 1.2; ambulatory= 1.3.
SF: stress factor. Minor surgery= 1.2; Trauma= 1.35; ARDS/Sepsis= 1.6; severe burn= 2.1.

http://www.medicalc.com/frmls/nutrition/**TEE.htm**

EEA Energy Expenditure of Activity **kcal/d**

Sedentary = 400 – 800
Light work = 800 – 1200
Moderate work = 1200 – 1800
Heavy work = 1800 – 4500

TEF Thermic Effect of Food **kcal/d**

TEF = 10% of BMR

(formerly called specific dynamic action of food)

http://www.medicalc.com/frmls/nutrition/**TEF.htm**

Nutritional Status

NB Nitrogen Balance

$$NB = \frac{\text{protein intake, g}}{6.25} - \frac{\text{UUN, g}}{0.8} + 2.0g^*$$

http://www.medicalc.com/frmls/nutrition/**NB.htm**

Zero = normal healthy

Negative = protein deficit (net catabolism)

Positive = growth and repair

* UUN/0.8 represents UUN plus urinary nonurea N+.
* 2g is the sum of fecal and integumental N+.

CatIndex Catabolic Index

CI = UUN, g – [(0.5 * protein intake*0.16) + 3.0g]

http://www.medicalc.com/frmls/nutrition/**CatIndex.htm**

normal = < 0.0

moderate nutritional stress from 0.0 to <5.0

severe nutritional stress > 5.0

* 3g is the sum of fecal and integumental N+.

Protein Nitrogen Content (avg protein is 16% N+)

grams protein = 6.25(grams of N+)

http://www.medicalc.com/frmls/nutrition/**PNC.htm**

TULN Total Urine Loss of Nitrogen **g**

TULN = (UUN * Urine Volume) / (0.8)

* UUN = ~80% of urinary nitrogen

http://www.medicalc.com/frmls/nutrition/**TULN.htm**

BUN <--> Urea conversion

BUN = Urea/2.14 Urea = BUN * 2.14

http://www.medicalc.com/frmls/nutrition/**BUNToUrea.htm**

Creatinine/Height ratio **> 95%**

> 9.5mg/cm. (Cr in g/d, height in cm).

IUCr Ideal Urinary Creatinine

M = IBW (kg) * 23 mg/kg

F = IBW (kg) * 18 mg/kg

---

* Protein intake/6.25 is equivalent to protein intake*0.16 (because protein ~ 16% N+)
* fecal and integumental N+ varies between 2 and 3 g per day.

Nutritional Status

PNI Prognostic Nutritional Index %

PNI= 158 – (16.6*Alb) – (0.78*TSF) – (0.2*TFN) – (5.8*DH-3 antigens)

Risk: Low = < 40%
Moderate = 40 – 49%
High = > 50%

http://www.medicalc.com/frmls/nutrition/**PNI.htm**

POS Probability of Survival %

POS= (0.91*Alb) – (1.0*DSH) – (1.44*SEP) + (0.98*DoC) –1.09

Alb= serum albumin.
DSH= delayed skin hypersensitivity (1=anergy, 2=reactive).
SEP= Sepsis (1= no sepsis, 2= sepsis).
DoC= Diagnosis of cancer (1= no cancer, 2= cancer).

http://www.medicalc.com/frmls/nutrition/**POS.htm**

Anthropometrics

ANTHROPOMETRIC ANALYSIS

Midarm muscle and adipose compartments:

MAC =	Mid upper Arm Circumference, in cm
TSF =	Triceps Skinold, in mm
MMC =	Midarm Muscle Circumference, in cm
MMA =	Midarm Muscle Area, in cm2
MFA =	Midarm Fat Area, in cm2
MA =	Midarm Area (total), in cm2

		M:	**F:**
MMC =	MAC – Π TSF	25.3cm	23.2cm
	http://www.medicalc.com/frmls/nutrition/**MMC.htm**		
MMA =	[(MAC – Π TSF)^2] /4Π	50.9cm2	42.8cm2
	http://www.medicalc.com/frmls/nutrition/**MMA.htm**		
MFA =	[(MAC*TSF)/2] – [Π(TSF^2)/4]	17cm2	21.3cm2
	http://www.medicalc.com/frmls/nutrition/**MFA.htm**		
MA =	Π * [(MAC/2)/Π]^2	57.9cm2	64.1cm2
	http://www.medicalc.com/frmls/nutrition/**MA.htm**		
TSF =	Direct measurement	12.5mm	16.5mm

MA= MFA + MMA. (MAC/2)/Π = diameter/2. (^2 denotes to the power of 2).

Calories

Caloric Content*

CHO (carbohydrates)	1g	=	4.0kcal
Lipids (fat) Long chain	1g	=	9.0kcal
medium chain	1g	=	7.1kcal
Proteins	1g	=	4.0kcal
dextrose	1g	=	3.4kcal
etOH	1g	=	7.0kcal

* represent average values.

Protein Requirements

Maintenance:

Normal	= 0.8 g protein/kg IBW/d
Stress (moderate)	= 1.0 – 1.5 g protein/kg IBW/d
Stress (severe)	= 2.0 – 2.6 g protein/kg IBW/d

Renal Failure:

ClCR >20mL/min	= 0.5 – 0.8 g protein/kg IBW/d
ClCR 10–20mL/min	= 0.5 g protein/kg IBW/d
Hemodialysis	= 1.0 – 1.2 g protein/kg IBW/d
Peritoneal dialysis	= 1.2 – 1.5 g protein/kg IBW/d

Anabolism:

requirements	= 1.0 – 1.5 g protein/kg IBW/d
BUN/Cr (S) ratio	= > 20 suggests overfeeding

Body Compartments

MASS & COMPOSITION OF BODY COMPARTMENTS

Protoplasm* = 50% of BW, (27g N+, 97mmol P & 150mEq K+)
ExtraCellular Fluid = 24% of BW, (140mEq Na+ & 96mEq Cl-)
Bone = 7% of BW, (260g Ca++ & 115g P)
Adipose Tissue = 19% of BW.

*per kg of dry wt

Δ Protoplasm (g)	= 27 * Δ N+ (g)
Δ ECF (g)	= 9.6 * Δ Cl- (mEq)
Δ Bone (g)	= 0.1 * Δ Ca++ (mEq)
Δ Adipose tissue (g)	= Δ BW (g) – (Δ protoplasm + ΔECF + Δbone)

adapted from REIFENSTEIN EC: J Clin Endocrinol Metab 5: 367, 1945

GASTROINTESTINAL

SAAG Serum/Ascitis Albumin Gradient **g/dL***

SAAG = albumin (S) – albumin (Ascitis)

http://www.medicalc.com/frmls/gastroint/**SAAG.htm**

gradient = > 1.1 g/dL in portal hypertension

Discriminant Function

DiscFctn = [(PTpt – PTcontrol) x (4.6)] + bilirubin

http://www.medicalc.com/frmls/gastroint/**DiscFctn.htm**

if > 32, Rx with steroids is recommended.

* PT = Prothrombin time. pt = patient.

*bilirubin in umol/L (If bilirubin in mg/dL, divide by 17).

SOURCE: NEJM, Feb 1992.

AST/ALT-r AST/ALT ratio

http://www.medicalc.com/frmls/gastroint/**ASTALT_r.htm**

If > 2 suggests alcoholic liver disease.

*AST= aspartate aminotransferase *ALT= alanine aminotransferase

SOG Stool Osmolar Gap **mOsm/kg**

SOG = measured Osm, stl – calculated Osm (stl)

http://www.medicalc.com/frmls/gastroint/**SOG.htm**

OsmStl stool Osmolality (calculated) **mOsm/kg**

OsmStl = 2 x [Na+ (stl) **+** K+ (stl)]

http://www.medicalc.com/frmls/gastroint/**OsmStl.htm**

Ascitis

ASCITIC FLUID:

protein	Ascitis/Serum	> 0.5 suggests malignancy
LDH		elevated in malignancy
CEA (mg/dL)		> 10.0 suggests malignancy
CEA	Ascitis/Serum	> 2.0 suggests malignancy
Amylase		elevated in "pancreatic ascitis"
Triglycerids		elevated in "chylous ascitis"

CELLS		
RBCs	>10,000/mm3	pancreatic ascitis, neoplasm.
	<10,000/mm3	nephrosis, any disease.
WBCs	>1,000/mm3	panc ascitis, neoplasm, TB
	<1,000/mm3	panc ascitis, CHF, cirrhosis,etc.
	PMN mainly	pyogenic peritonitis.

ENDOCRINE

Cholesterol

LDL Low Density Lipoprotein cholesterol **60-130mg/dL***

$$LDL = cholesterol - \left(\frac{TG}{5} + HDL \right)$$

http://www.medicalc.com/frmls/endo/**LDL.htm**

(if mmol/L) LDL = cholesterol – (TG/2.2 + HDL)

VLDL Very Low Density Lipoprotein **12-32mg/dL***

VLDL = TG/5

http://www.medicalc.com/frmls/endo/**VLDL.htm**

CholHDL-r Cholesterol/HDL ratio **< 5**

(the lower the better).

LDL/HDL-r LDL/HDL ratio **< 3**

* Depends on risk factors and Rx goals, see NCEP guidelines and summary of the 2nd Report (JAMA 269:3015,1993)
* HDL= high density lipoproteins. TG= triglycerids.
* all values in (P, S) mg/dL.

Insulin

Insulin/Glucose ratio Insulin uU/mL; glucose mg/dL

nl = < 0.4

insulinoma = > 0.4 (often > 1.0)

* values in P or S.

Thyroid

FT4I Free Thyroxine Index **1.2 – 5.0**

FT4I = T3RU (%) * T4

FT3I Free Triiodothyronine Index

FT3I = T3RU (%) * T3

* T3RU = Triiodothyronine resin uptake.
* FT3I and FT4I en % terms.

PEDIATRICS

* mm ID= milimeters of internal diameter.

TubeSize1 **mm ID***

$$\text{TubeSize}^* = \frac{\text{age (yr)}}{4.0} + (4.0)$$

http://www.medicalc.com/frmls/peds/**TubeSize1.htm**

TubeSize2 **mm ID***

$$\text{TubeSize}^* = \frac{16 + \text{age (yr)}}{4.0}$$

http://www.medicalc.com/frmls/peds/**TubeSize2.htm**

ETT_e estimation of EndoTracheal Tube **mm ID***

$$\text{TubeSize}^* = \frac{\text{postconceptual age (wks)}}{10}$$

http://www.medicalc.com/frmls/peds/**ETT_e.htm**

Dist4Ins distance for insertion of ETT **cm**

$$\text{Distance (cm)} = \frac{\text{age (yr)}}{2.0} + (12.0)$$

http://www.medicalc.com/frmls/peds/**Dist4Ins.htm**

SBPped median Systolic Blood Pressure* **mmHg**

SBP = 90 mmHg + (2 x age in years)

http://www.medicalc.com/frmls/peds/**SBPped.htm**

* for children older than 1 year.

H2OlossU Urinary water losses **mL**

H2OlossU = 60 mL/kg/day

http://www.medicalc.com/frmls/peds/**H2OlossU.htm**

H2OlossF Fecal water losses **mL**

H2OlossF = 10 mL/kg/day

http://www.medicalc.com/frmls/peds/**H2OlossF.htm**

H2OlossIns Insensible water losses **mL**

H2OlossIns = 30 mL/kg/day

http://www.medicalc.com/frmls/peds/**H2OlossIns.htm**

* each celsius degree ↑ in temperature (>37.2) ↑ insensible water losses by 7 mL/kg/24h.

---

*all values and formulas for pediatric patients (water losses may vary substantially).

HEMATOLOGY

Fe++ def Iron Deficit **0 mg**

Fe def = [Wt * (15 – Hb)] + 1000

http://www.medicalc.com/frmls/hemato/**Fe_def.htm**

* 15 is the normal Hb (hemoglobin). * Wt in Lb. Hb in g/dL

TransFe Transferrin **220-400mg/dL**

TransFe = (0.8 * TIBC) – 43

http://www.medicalc.com/frmls/hemato/**TransFe.htm**

* TIBC = total iron binding capacity (ug/dL)

INR International Normalized Ratio **2.0 – 3.0**

INR = (PT patient/PT control)^ISI

* PT = Prothrombin time. pt = patient.

Cells

ANC Absolute Neutrophil Count **$1x10^3/mm^3$**

ANC = WBC * [(PMN/100) + (bands/100)]

http://www.medicalc.com/frmls/hemato/**ANC.htm**

* WBC= white blood cells, PMN= polymorphonuclear cells.

ARC Absolute Reticulocyte Count **cells/L**

$$ARC = \frac{\text{Retis \%}}{100} \times \text{RBC count } (x10^{12}/L)$$

http://www.medicalc.com/frmls/hemato/**ARC.htm**

Retic_c Corrected Reticulocytes **%**

$$Retic\_c = \text{Retis \%} \times \frac{\text{(Hct Patient)}}{\text{Hct Normal}}$$

http://www.medicalc.com/frmls/hemato/**Retic_c.htm**

* Hct = hematocrit (mL/dL). Normal Hct = 45.

Retic_pc percentage of Reticulocytes* **%**

$$Retic\_pc = \frac{\text{number of Retis}}{\text{RBC observed}} \times 100$$

http://www.medicalc.com/frmls/hemato/**Retic_pc.htm**

* usually based on 1000 RBC count.

CSF					
	Appearance	***Glucose*** (mg/dL)	***Protein*** (mg/dL)	***Pressure*** (mmHg)	***Cell count*** (cell/mm^3)
Normal	clear	50-80	20-45	100-200	<6 Lymphs
Meningitis:					
acute bacterial	cloudy	↓↓	↑↑	↑↑	↑↑, PMN
aseptic (viral)	clear/cloudy	N	↑	N / ↑	↑, Monos
TB meningitis	cloudy	↓	↑	↑	↑, PMN (early)
Fungal	clear/cloudy	↓	↑	↓	↑ Monocytes
Hemorrhage	bloody/ xanto*	N / ↓	↑	↑	↑↑ , RBC
Neoplasm	clear / xanto*	N / ↓	N / ↑	↑↑	N / ↑ Lymphs
Neurosyphilis	clear/cloudy	N	↑	N / ↑	↑ Monocytes
Guilain-Barré	clear/cloudy	N	↑↑	N	N / ↑ Lymphs

*CSF = cerebrospinal fluid. PMN= polymorphonuclear cells. xanto= xantochromia

PLEURAL FLUID

PLEURAL FLUID

TEST	Transudate	Exudate
LDH (IU/dL)	<200	>200 (high)
fluid/serum ratio	<0.6	>0.6
Proteins	<3.0g/dL	>3.0g/dL
fluid/serum ratio	<0.5	>0.5
Specific gravity	<1.016	>1.016
WBC's	<1,000/uL	>1,000/uL >50%lymphs:TB,CA >50%PMN: inflam.
RBC's	<10,000/uL	<100,000/uL(?)
Amylase	---	>500 (pancreatitis)
Glucose	same as blood	low (<60mg/dL) (<10-20 = RA)
pH	>7.3	<7.3

*CA= cancer. TB= tuberculosis. RA= rheumatoid arthritis.
PMN= polymorphonuclear cells.

SYNOVIAL FLUID

SYNOVIAL FLUID

Condition = color, clarity, WBC/mm3, PMN

Normal = colorless, transparent, <200 WBC, <25%PMN

NonInflammatory= straw, transparent, 200-2000 WBC, <25% PMN
(osteoarthritis, trauma, SLE, aseptic necrosis)

Inflammatory= Yellow, translucent, 2,000-75,000 WBC, 40-75% PMN
RA, gout, pseudogout, SLE, SSA.

Septic = variable, opaque, >75,000 WBC, >75% PMN
bacterial infection, TB

*RA = rheumatoid arthritis. SLE= systemic lupus erythematosus.
*SSA= seronegative spondyloarthropathies.
*WBC/mm3.
*culture may be + in septic, crystals may be present in Inflammatory.

STATISTICS

Sensitivity = Probability that the test/procedure will be positive when the disease is present.

True positive rate = sensitivity %

False negative rate (100 – sensitivity) = Probability that the test/procedure will be negative when the disease is present.

Specificity = Probability that the test/procedure will be negative when the disease is not present.

True negative rate = specificity %

False positive rate (100 – specificity)

Positive Predictive Value = Probability that disease is present when test/procedure is positive.

Negative Predictive Value = Probability that disease is not present when test/procedure is negative.

GOLD STANDARD

		Disease State	
		Present	Absent
TEST RESULT	positive +	true positive **a**	false positive **b**
	– negative	**c** false negative	**d** true negative

Sensitivity = a / (a + c)
Specificity = d / (b + d)
Positive Predictive Value = a / (a + b)
Negative Predictive Value = d / (c + d)
False-Negative Rate = c / (a + c)
False-Positive Rate = b (b + d)
Accuracy (overall) = (a + d) / (a + d + c + d)
Prevalence = (a + c) / (a + b + c + d)

Normal Values

Blood Chemistry

TEST	specimen	Value Units
Acetoacetate	P	0.2-1.0mg/dL
AFP	S	mg/dL
Albumin,	S	3.5-5.5g/dL
ALT (SGPT)	S	0-35U/L
AST (SGOT)	S	0-35U/L
Ammonia	P	20-120ug/dL
Amylase	S	60-180U/dL
Anion Gap		8-12mEq/L
Base, total	S	145-155mEq/L
Bilirubin, total	S	0.3-1.0mg/dL
direct		0.1-0.3mg/dL
indirect		0.2-0.7mg/dL
BUN	S	10-20mg/dL
Calcium, total	P	9.0-10.5mg/dL
ionized		4.5-5.6mg/dL
		46-50% of total
CEA	S	0 - 2.5ng/mL
smoker		0-5.0ng/mL
Chloride	S	98-106mEq/L
Cholesterol	S	<200mg/dL
LDL		<130mg/dL
HDL		27-98mg/dL
Cortisol	P	5-23ug/d (AM)
		3-15ug/d (PM)
CO2 content	P	22-31mmol/L
CPK	S	25-90U/mL
CPK MB		<3% - 5%
Creatinine	S	<1.5mg/dL
Ferritin	S	10-400ng/mL
GGT	S	12-76IU/L
Globulin	S	2.0-3.5g/dL

*SGPT = serum glutamic pyruvic transaminase. SGOT= serum glutamic oxalacetic t.

Blood Chemistry

TEST	specimen	Value Units
Glucose	B	60-100mg/dL
Hemoglobin a1c		< 6% (tot Hb)
Iron, total	S	70-140mg/dL
TIBC		273-337ug/dL
%sat		20-45%
Ketones, total	S	0.5-1.5mg/dL
LDH	S	90-280IU/L
Lead	S	<20ug/dL
Lipase	S	2.3-20IU/dL
Magnesium	S	2.0-3.0mg/dL
Osmolality	S	275-295mos/kg
Phosphatase	S	
Acid: total:		0-0.7IU/L
Prostatic		<3.0ng/mL
Alkaline	S	38-126IU/L
Phosphate	S	3.0-4.5mg/dL
Potassium	S	3.5-5.0mEq/L
Prealbumin	S	10-40mg/dL
Protein, tot	S	5.5-8.0g/dL
PSA	S	<4.0ng/mL
Sodium	S	136-145mEq/L
Thyroid: TT4	S	5-12ug/dL
Free T4		0.8-2.4ng/dL
T3		115-190ng/dL
T3 uptake		25-35%
TSH		2-10uIU/dL
Transferrin	S	220-400mg/dL
Triglycerides	P	<250mg/dL
Uric acid	S	2.5-8.0mg/dL
Vit B12	S	200-800pg/mL
Zinc	S	11.5-18.5ug/dL

* P= plasma. S= serum.

Hematology

TEST	specimen	Value Units
Hematocrit	B	M: 42-52mL/dL F: 37-47mL/dL
Hemoglobin	B	M: 14-18g/dL F: 12-16g/dL
RBC's	B	M:5.4±0.9x10^6/uL F: 4.8±0.6x10^6/uL
MCV		90±7fL
MCH		29±2pg/cell
MCHC		34±2g/dL
RDW		11.8-14.6%
Reticulocytes		0.5-1.5%
WBC's total	B	3.8-9. 8x10^3 /uL
Segmented		40-60%
Bands		0-5%
Lymphocytes		20-40%
Mononuclear		4-8%
Eosinophils		1-3%
Basophils		0-1%
Platelets	B	190-405x10^3/uL
Lymphocyte (differential)		
B cell		5-25%
T cell		60-88%
Suppressor (CD8)		10-43%
Helper (CD4)		32-66%
H : S (ratio)		1.0

* B= whole blood. P= plasma. S= serum. F = female. M = male.

Hematology NORMAL VALUES

TEST	specimen	Value Units
Antithrombin III		21-30mg/dL
Bleeding time		2-7min (<9min)
Carboxy-Hb	B	0-2.3% of tot Hb
Clot retraction	B	begind at 1h, usually 6h, complete at 24h (appreciative test).
Clotting time	B	5-8min
ESR	B	M: 0-9mm/h F: 0-20mm/h
Fibrinogen	P	200-400mg/dL
FDP's	P	<10ug/mL
Haptoglobin	S	83-267mg/dL
LAP		13-100Umg/dL
Met Hb	B	0.78±0.37% of total
Platelets		
Count	B	290,000/uL
Aggregation	P	full response to ADP, epinephrine, collagen.
Factor III	P	33-57s
Prothrombin Time (PT)	B	11-15s (VII)
Protein C	P	<5ug/mL
Protein S	P	<5ug/mL
PT	B	11-15s (VII)
aPTT	B	20-35s (XII, XI, IX, VIII)
Thrombin Time	B	control ± 2s (when control is 9-13s)
Viscosity	P	1.7-2.1 (H_2O)

* B= whole blood. P= plasma. S= serum. F = female. M = male.

Urine

TEST	Value Units
Albumin	<150mg/24h
Anion Gap	(Na + K - Cl)
δ-Aminolevulinic acid	1.3-1.7mg/d
Ammonia nitrogen	30-50mEq/d
Amylase	35-260U/h
Bilirubin	negative
Blood, occult	negative
Calcium, total	0-250mg/24h
Chloride	110-250mmol/d
Catecholamines	<540ug/d
Dopamine	<85ug/d
Epinephrine	0-13ug/d
Norepinephrine	11-86ug/d
Chloride	110-250mmol/d
Copper	15-50ug/d
Cortisol, free	20-90ug/d
Creatinine	M: 1.0-2.0g/d F: 0.6-1.5g/d
Fat	negative
FDP	<0.25ug/mL
Fructose	30 – 65mg/24h
GFR	125mL/min
Glucose	50-300mg/d
Hemoglobin	negative
HVA	<15mg/d
5-HIAA	0.2-5.7mg/d
17-OH	2-10mg/d
17-Ketos	M: 8-22mg/d F: 6-15mg/d
Ketones, total	50.5±30.7mg/dL
LDH	560-2050Units/8h
Lead	<120ug/d

* U = urine. F = female. M = male.

TEST	Value Units
Magnesium	6.0–8.5mEq/24h
Mercury	<20ug/L
Osmolality	50-1400mOsmol/kg
12h fluid rest	>850mOsmol/kg/d
Oxalate	8-40ug/d
Pentoses	2.0–5.0mg/kg/24h
Phosphorus	0.4-1.3g/d
Porphyrins, Uro-	0-27ug/d
Copro-	0-72ug/d
Potassium	25-100mEq/d
Protein, total	1-14mg/dL
Sodium	40-220mEq/d
Solids, total	55-70g/d
Specific gravity	
random urine	1.002-1.030
U, 12h fluid restriction	>1.025
U, 24h	1.015 – 1.025
Urea nitrogen	6-17g/24h
Uric acid	250-750mg/d
Urobilinogen	1.0-3.5mg/d
VMA	2-10mg/d
Volume	
total	600-2500mL/d
day/night ratio	4:1 to 2:1
Night volume	<700mL (SpGr >1.018)
Urine production rate	1mL/min
GFR	125mL/min
Zinc	0.15–1.2mg/24h

* U = urine. F = female. M = male.

*See notice about normal values in page X.

UNITS

SI Prefixes

SI = système international d'Unitès

10^{18}	exa	E	10^{-1}	deci	d
10^{15}	peta	P	10^{-2}	centi	c
10^{12}	tera	T	10^{-3}	mili	m
10^{9}	giga	G	10^{-6}	micro	μ (u)
10^{6}	mega	M	10^{-9}	nano	n
10^{3}	kilo	k	10^{-12}	pico	p
10^{2}	hecto	h	10^{-15}	femto	f
10^{1}	deka	da	10^{-18}	atto	a

SI Base Units

Quantity	Name of Unit	Symbol of units	Derivation of units (decimals)
SI Base Units			
Length	meter	m	
Mass	kilogram	kg	
Time	second	s	
Thermodynamic temperature	Kelvin	K	
Amount of substance	mole	mol	
Electric current	ampere	A	
Luminous intensity	candela	cd	

SI Derived Units UNITS

Quantity	Name of Unit	Symbol of units	Derived units (decimals)
SI Derived Units			
Area	square meter	m2	cm2, mm2
Volume	liter	L	mL, uL
Number	Unity	1	
Catalytic activity	katal	z	
Mass concentration	ρ	kg per liter	kg/L
Mass fraction	ϖ	kg/kg	
Volume fraction		L/L	mL/L
Substance concentration	c	mole/L	mmol/L, umol/L
Molality	m	mole/kg	mol/kg
Substance fraction	x	mole/mole	mmol/mmol
Number concentration	C	one/L	1/L
Celsius temperature	degree Celsius	°C	K
Force	newton	N	(m • kg)/s2
Pressure	pascal	Pa	N • m2
Partial Pressure	Newton/m2	N/m2	
Mass density	kg/L	kg/L	mg/L, mg/mL
Work, energy	joule	J	N • m

OTHER UNITS

Time	minute hour	min h	day year	d y

* SOURCE: adapted from RODRIGUEZ AA, *Medi-Data*, 3rd ED, 1995

CONVERSION

Conversions

LENGTH

1 inch	= 2.54cm	1cm	= 0.3937in
1 inch	= 25.4mm	1mm	= 0.03937in
1 foot	= 30.48cm	1m	= 3.28ft
1 yard	= 91.44cm	1m	= 1.093yd
1 mile	= 1609.3m	1km	= 1093.6yd
1m	= 100cm	1cm	= 0.01m
1cm	= 10mm	1mm	= 0.1cm

http://www.medicalc.com/frmls/conversion/**length.htm**

VOLUME

1 gallon	= 3.785 L	1L	= 0.264gal
1 fl oz	= 29.57mL	1mL	= 0.034fl oz
1L	= 1000mL	1mL	= 0.001L
1mL	= 1000uL	1uL	= 0.001mL

http://www.medicalc.com/frmls/conversion/**volume.htm**

TEMPERATURE

°F = (°C x 1.8) + 32

°C = (°F – 32)/1.8

°F =	°C	°F =	°C
90.4	33.0	99.5	37.5
91.3	33.5	100.4	38.0
92.2	34.0	101.3	38.5
93.1	34.5	102.2	39.0
94.0	35.0	103.1	39.5
95.9	35.5	104.0	40.0
96.8	36.0	104.9	40.5
97.7	36.5	105.8	41.0
98.6	37.0	106.7	41.5

http://www.medicalc.com/frmls/conversion/**temp.htm**

CONVERSION

MASS

1 grain	= 0.065g	1g	= 15.43grain
1 lb	= 0.454g		
1 Kg	= 2.2046 lb	1lb	= 0.4536kg

http://www.medicalc.com/frmls/conversion/**mass.htm**

CHEMICAL

$$\text{mEq/L} = \frac{\text{mg/dL} * 10 * \text{valence}}{\text{atomic weight}}$$

$$\text{mg/dL} = \frac{\text{mEq/L} * \text{atomic weight}}{10 * \text{valence}}$$

**in case of gases: Vol% x 10/22.4 = mmol/L (for CO_2 use 22.26)

http://www.medicalc.com/frmls/conversion/**mEqLTomgdL.htm**

PRESSURE

mmHg = cmH_2O * 1.36	1mmHg = 1.36cmH_2O
cmH_2O = mmHg * 0.732	1cmH_2O = 0.732mmHg

http://www.medicalc.com/frmls/conversion/**pressure.htm**

HOUSEHOLD MEASURES

1 teaspoonful = 0.17fl oz
1 dessertspoonful = 0.27fl oz
1 tablespoonful = 0.5fl oz
1 jigger = 1.5fl oz

1 wineglassful = 2.0fl oz
1 teacupful = 4.0fl oz
1 glassful = 8.0fl oz

http://www.medicalc.com/frmls/conversion/**household.htm**

gtt & microgtt

**(gtt = drop   micro gtt = micro drop)

1mL = 20 macrodrops (regular drops)
1mL = 60 microdrops (if using microtubing)

http://www.medicalc.com/frmls/conversion/**gtt.htm**

ABBREVIATIONS

A	adult
a	arterial
A-aDO2	Alveolar-arterial O2 Gradient
A Fib	atrial fibrillation
aB	arterial Blood
ABG	arterial blood gases
ABW	Adjusted Body Weight
ac	acute
AF	Activity Factor
AG	Anion Gap
AIVR	accelerated idioventricular rhythm
ALT	Alanine aminotransferase
AmCr_CI	Amylase/Creatinine Clearance ratio
ANC	Absolute Neutrophil Count
APD	atrial premature depolarization
ARC	Absolute Reticulocyte Count
AST	Aspartate aminotransferase
B	whole blood
BEE	Basal Energy Expenditure
BFVR	Blood Flow Volume Ratio
BMI	Body Mass Index
BMR	Basal Metabolic Rate
BP, SAP	Blood pressure
bpm	beats per minute
BSA	Body surface area
BV	Blood Volume
BW	body weight
c	capillary
C(a-v)O2	arterial - venous O2 content difference
C.O.	cardiac output
Ca_pb	protein-bound Calcium
CaCO2	arterial CO2 content
CaO2	arterial O2 content
CBF	Cerebral Blood Flow
CBVI	Central Blood Volume Index
CC	Closing Capacity
CC/TLC	closing capacity/total lung capacity
CcO2	capillary O2 content
cd	candela
Cdyn	Dynamic Compliance
CEA	carcinoembryonic antigen

ABBREVIATIONS

CH	children
CHO	Carbohydrates
CholHDL-r	Cholesterol/HDL ratio
CI	Cardiac Index
Cl	clearance
Cl- def	Chloride Deficit
Cl H_2O	Free Water Clearance
Cl Osm	Osmolar Clearance
Cl PAH	p-Aminohippurate Clearance
Cl Urea	Urea Clearance
ClCr	Creatinine Clearance
cm	centimeter
CO	Cardiac Output
conc	concentration
COP	Colloid-Oncotic Pressure
COPD	chronic obstructive pulmonary disease
Cr	creatinine
CSF	cerebrospinal fluid
Cspec	Specific Compliance
Cstat	Static Compliance ($\Delta V/\Delta P$)
CV	Closing Volume
CV/VC	closing volume/vital capacity
CvO_2	mixed venous O2 content
CVP	Central venous pressure
d	day
Δ	change
DO_2	Oxygen Delivery
DO_2I	Oxygen Delivery Index
DW	dextrose water
ECF	Extracellular fluid
ECG	Electrocardiogram
EDV	End-Diastolic Volume
EE	Energy Expenditure
EEA	Energy Expenditure of Activity
EF	Ejection Fraction
ERV	Expiratory Reserve Volume
ESV	End-Systolic Volume
etOH	ethanol
ETT_e	endotracheal tube estimation
F	female
FE Urea	fractional excretion of Urea

Abbreviations

FE Uric a	fractional excretion of Uric acid
Fe++ def	Iron Deficit
$FEF_{200-1200}$	Forced Expiratory Flow
FEF_{25-75}	Forced Mid-Expiratory Flow
$FEF_{50\%}$	Forced Expiratory Flow at 50%
$FEF_{75\%}$	Forced Expiratory Flow at 75%
FEK+	Fractional Excretion of K+*
FENa+	fractional excretion of Sodium
F_EO_2	Fraction of Expired O2
FEPi	Fractional Excretion of Pi*
FEVz	Forced Expiratory Volume at z
FIF_{25-75}	Forced Mid-Inspiratory Flow
F_IO_2	Fraction of Inspired O2
fl oz	fluid ounce
FRC	Functional Residual Capacity
frm	formula
ft	foot
FT_3I	Free Triiodothyronine Index
FT_4I	Free Thyroxine Index
FVC	Forced Vital Capacity
gal	gallon
G_{aw}	Airway Conductance at FRC
GFR	Glomerular filtration rate, estimated
gn	grain
gtt	drop
h	hour
H+	Hydrogen, acid
H+ def	Acid deficit
H2Oloss	water loss
H_2O_xs	Free Water excess
Hb	hemoglobin
HCO_3	bicarbonate
HCO_3 def	Bicarbonate deficit
Hct	hematocrit
HR	Heart Rate
IBW	Ideal Body Weight
IBW%	percentage of IBW
IC	Inspiratory Capacity
ICF	Intracellular fluid
IM	Intramuscular
in	inch
INR	International Normalized Ratio

ABBREVIATIONS

IRV	Inspiratory Reserve Volume
IUCr	Ideal Urinary Creatinine
IV	Intravascular fluid
IV	Intravenously
K	Kelvin
K+	Potassium
K+ def	Potassium Deficit
kg	kilogram
L	Liter
L_xs	Lactate excess
LAD	left anterior descending
LAH	left atrial hypertrophy
LBBB	left bundle branch block
LBM	Lean Body Mass
LCWI	Left Cardiac Work Index
LDH	Lactate dehydrogenase
LDL/HDL-r	LDL/HDL ratio
LDLc	Low Density Lipoprotein cholesterol
LVH	left ventricular hypertrophy
LVSWI	Left Vent Stroke Work Index
m	meter
M	male
MAC	Mid upper Arm Circumference
MAP	Mean Arterial Pressure
MAT	multifocal atrial tachycardia
MBF	Myocardial Blood Flow
MEP	Maximal Expiratory Pressure
MFA	Midarm Fat Area
mi	mile
MIF	Maximal Inspiratory Force
min	minute
MIP	Maximal Inspiratory Pressure
mL	mililiter
MMA	Midarm Muscle Area
MMC	Midarm Muscle Circumference
mol	mole
MPAP	Mean Pulmonary Arterial Press.
MTT	Mean Transit Time
MVV	Maximal Voluntary Ventilation
Na+ def	Sodium Deficit
NB	Nitrogen Balance

Abbreviations

$NH4+$	ammonia
NIF	negative inspiratory force
nl (Nl)	normal
NS	normal saline
NSR	Normal sinus rhythm
O_2 ext	Oxygen extraction rate
°	degree
Osm	Osmolality
OTRCF	O2 Transport /Red Cell Flow ratio
OTRCM	O2 Transport /Red Cell mass ratio
P	plasma
$P(A\text{-}a)O_2$	Alveolar-arterial O2 difference (gradient)
P50	PaO2 at which Hb is 50% saturated
$PaCO_2$	arterial CO2 tension
$PACO_2$	alveolar CO2 tension
$PaCO_2$	arterial CO2 tension
PaO_2	arterial O2 tension
PAO_2	alveolar O2 tension
PAOP	pulmonary artery oclussion pressure
PAP	Pulmonary arterial pressure
PAT	paroxysmal atrial tachycardia
P_B	Barometric pressure
PE	pulmonary embolism
P_ECO_2	expired CO2 tension
PEEP	Positive End-Expiratory Pressure
pH	potential hydrogen
PH_2O	Water vapor pressure
P_IO_2	Inspired O2 tension
PNI	Prognostic Nutritional Index
PO	oral (oral route)
POS	Probability of Survival
PP	Pulse Pressure
prn	pro re nata (as needed)
P_{st} TLC	Static Recoil Pressure at TLC
Pt	patient
PT	Prothrombin time
PV	Plasma volume
PVC	premature ventricular depolarization
$PvCO_2$	mixed venous CO2 tension
PvO_2	mixed venous O2 tension
PVR	Pulmonary Vascular Resistance
PVRI	Pulmonary Vasc Resist Index

ABBREVIATIONS

q	every
qd	every day
qh	every hour
QRS	QRS segment
QS	Shunted Blood R → L
QS/QT	Shunt Fraction R → L
QT	Pulmonary Blood Flow
R	Respiratory Quotient
RAH	right atrial hypertrophy
Raw	Airway Resistance
RBBB	right bundle branch block
RBC	red blood cell
RBF	Renal Blood Flow, basal
RCA	right coronary artery
RCFR	Red Cell Flow Rate
RCV	Red cell volume
RCWI	Right Cardiac Work Index
Retic_c	Corrected Reticulocytes
Retic_pc	percentage of Reticulocytes
RFI	renal failure index
RL	Pulmonary Resistance at FRC
RL	ringer lactated
RPP	Rate Pressure Product
RR	Respiratory rate
RTA	renal tubular acidosis
RV	Residual Volume
RV/TLC	residual volume/total lung capacity
RVH	right ventricular hypertrophy
RVI	right ventricle infarction
RVSWI	Right vent stroke work index
S	serum
s	second
SAAG	Serum/Ascitis Albumin Gradient
SaO2	Arterial O2 saturation
SAP	Systemic arterial pressure
SBPped	SBP for pediatrics
SC	subcutaneously
ScO2	capillary O2 saturation
SF	Stress Factor
sp gr	specific gravity
SV	Stroke Volume

Abbreviations

SVI	Stroke Volume Index
SvO_2	Mixed Venous O2 saturation
SVR	Systemic Vascular Resistance
SVRI	Systemic Vascular Resistance Index
SVT	supraventricular tachycardia
T	Temperature
TBS	Total Body Solute
TBW	Total Body Water
TEE	Total Energy Expenditure
TEF	Thermic Effect of Food
TLC	Total Lung Capacity
TOEE	Tissue O2 Extraction Efficiency
TOEI	Tissue O2 Extraction Index
TransFe	Transferrin
TRP	Tubular Reabsorption of Phosphate
TSF	Triceps Skinold
TTKG	Transtubular Potassium Gradient
TULN	Total Urine Loss of Nitrogen
TV	Tidal Volume
U	unit
U	urine
U24h	24h urine
UaCr_r	Uric acid / creatinine ratio
v	venous
V Fib	ventricular fibrillation
V Tach	ventricular tachycardia
V_A	Alveolar Volume
V_A	Alveolar Ventilation
V_A/Q	VA/Blood Flow
vB	venous blood
VC	Vital Capacity
VCO_2	Carbon Dioxide Output
V_D	Volume of Dead Space
V_D	Dead Space Ventilation
V_D/V_T	Dead Space/Tidal volume ratio
V_E	Minute Ventilation
VLDL	Very Low Density Lipoprotein
VO_2	Oxygen Consumption
VO_2I	Oxygen Consumption Index
vol	volume
VPD	ventricular premature depolarization

ABBREVIATIONS

W	Work of quiet Breathing
wk	week
W_{max}	Maximal Work of Breathing
WP	Wedge pressure
y	year
yd	yard

INTERNET and WWW

The ▶ icon indicates the internet address of the formula.

analog	any representation of info in which the amount of signal is proportional to the info represented.
applet	small piece of executable code written in JAVA that runs on the browser
apps	applications
bit	binary digit
bps	bits per second
client	a computer program that uses the internet to contact a remote server.
digital	technology that uses numbers to represent information
DNS	domain name system
domain name	the name assigned to a computer on the internet
ftp	file transfer protocol
htm	suffix of an internet document (also html)
HTML	hypertext markup language
http	hypertext transport protocol
hyperlinks	
hypertext	system for page storage of text information that contains references to other pages.
modem	modulator-demodulator, device used for the transmission of data across an analog path.
www	world wide web

REFERENCES

ADROGUE HJ, MADIAS NE: Changes in plasma potassium concentration during acute acid-base disturbances, Am J Med 71: 456, 1981

ADROGUE HJ, MADIAS NE: Medical Progress: Management of Life threatening Acid-Base Disorders. (I of II) NEJM 338: 26, 1998

ADROGUE HJ, MADIAS NE: Medical Progress: Management of Life threatening Acid-Base Disorders. (II of II) NEJM 338: 107, 1998

ALTMAN PL (Ed): Blood and other Body Fluids. Federation of American Societies for Experimental Biology, Washington, 1961

BERNARD J: Todd-Sanford-Davishon: Clinical Diagnosis and Management by Laboratory Methods, 17th ED, Philadelphia, WB Saunders, 1984

BOYD JR (Editor): Facts and Comparisons. J.B Lippincott Co. St. Louis 1984

BLACKBURN GL, et al: Nutritional and Metabolic Assessment of the Hospitalized Patient, JPEN 1: 11 1977

BRAUNWALD E: Heart Disease: A Textbook of Cardiovascular Medicine, 2nd ED, Philadelphia, WB Saunders, 1984

BRENNER BM, RECTOR FC: The Kidney, 3rd ED, Philadelphia, WB Saunders, 1986

COCKCROFT DW, GAULT MH: Prediction of Creatinine Clearance from Serum Creatinine, Nephron 16: 31-41, 1976

COHEN JJ, KASSIRER JP: Acid-Base. Boston, Little, Brown and Co, 1982

COLTON T: Statistics in Medicine, Little, Brown and Co. Boston 1974

COOKSEY FD: Clinical Vectorcardiography and Electrocardiography, 2nd ED, Year Book Medical Publishers, Chicago 1977

DIBKAER R: International Union of Pure and Applied Chemistry and International Federation of Clinical Chemistry: Approved Recommendation (1978). Quantities and Units in Clinical Chemistry. Clin Chim Acta, 96: 185F, 1979

Dig Dis Sci 24: 835, 1979.

Discriminant Function, NEJM Feb 1992.

DUBIN D: Rapid Interpretation of the EKG's, 3rd ED, Cover Publishing, 1974

EMMETT M, NARINS GR: Clinical Use of the Anion Gap, Medicine 56: 1594, 1976

References

ESPINEL CH, GREGORY AW: Differential Diagnosis of Acute Renal Failure, Clin Neph 13: 73, 1980

ESPINEL CH: The FENa+ Test, JAMA 236: 579, 1976

EWALD GA, McKENZIE CR (Eds): The Washington Manual, Manual of Medical Therapeutics, 28th ED, Boston, Little Brown & Co, 1995

FISHMAN AP (ED): Pulmonary Diseases and Disorders, 2nd ED, New York McGraw Hill Book Company, 1987

GABOW PA, et al: Diagnostic importance of an increased serum anion gap, NEJM 303: 854, 1980

GOODMAN A: Goodman & Gilman's: The Pharmacological Basis of Therapeutics, McMillan Publishing Company, 1985

GUYTON AC: Textbook of Medical Physiology, WB Saunders, Philadelphia 1983

HAYNES RB: How to read Clinical Journals: II To leran about a Diagnostic Test, Can Med Assoc J 1981; 124: 703-710

HUMES DH, NARINS GR, BRENNER BM: Disorders of Water balance, Hosp Prac, March 1979

ISSELBACHER KJ: Harrison's Principles of Internal Medicine, 14th ED, New York, McGraw Hill Book Company, 1994

Kidney Int 27: 472, 1985

Lancet, APR 1977 p785, Editorial: The Anion Gap

LEVINE RI, et al: Enhancement of the amylase/creatinine clearance ratio in disorders other than Acute Pancreatitis, NEJM 292:329, 1975

NARINS RG, et al: Lactic Acidosis and the elevated anion gap (I & II) Hosp Prac, May and June, 1980

NARINS RG, et al: Diagnostic Strategies in Disorders of Fluid, electrolyte and Acid-Base homeostasis, Am J Med: 496, 1982

NARINS GR, EMMETT M: Simple and Mixed Acid Base Disorders: A Practical Approach, Medicine, 59: 161, 1980

PERLMUTTER M: Urine-Serum Urea Nitrogen Ratio, JAMA 170:1533, 1959

REIFENSTEIN EC: J Clin Endocrinol Metab 5: 367, 1945

References

ROBINSON AG, LOEB JN: Ethanol ingestion commonest cause of elevated plasma osmolality? NEJM 284: 1253, 1971

RODRIGUEZ AA (Ed): *Medi*Formulas™ "The Medical Formulas & Equations" , 1st Ed, Rodram Corp, Mexico City, 1998

RODRIGUEZ AA (Ed): Medi-Data "Normal Values", 3rd Ed, Rodram Corp, Mexico City, 1995

RUBENSTEIN E: Scientific American Medicine, Scientific American, New York 1984

SCHRIER RW: Renal and Electrolyte Disorders, Little Brown & Company Boston 1983

SCULLY RE: Case Records of the Massachusetts General Hospital: Normal Reference Laboratory Values. N Engl J Med 314: 39-47, 1986

SHOEMAKER WC: Textbook of Critical Care, 1st ED, Philadelphia, WB Saunders 1985

SLEISINGER MH, FORDTRAN JS: Gastrointestinal Disease, 3rd ED Philadelphia, WB Saunders 1983

STEDMAN'S Medical Dictionary, 25th ED, Williams & Wilkins, Baltimore 1990

WEST JB: Pulmonary Pathophysiology: The essentials, Williams & Wilkins Baltimore, 1977

WILLIAMS WJ: Hematology, 3rd ED, New York, McGraw Hill, 1983

WINTROBE MM: Clinical Hematology, 8th ED Philadelphia, WB Saunders 1981

WYNGAARDEN JB (Ed): Cecil Textbook of Medicine, 17th Ed. Philadelphia WB Saunders Company, 1985

World Health Organization: Use of "Systeme International" in Medicine WHO official records No. 240, p21, 1977, Geneva, Switzerland

ALPHABETIC INDEX

A

Index

B

C

INDEX

D

Index

G

H

I

Index

Index

Q R

Index

S

T

I7hT YG13AW Y23HW